A woman's guide to sex

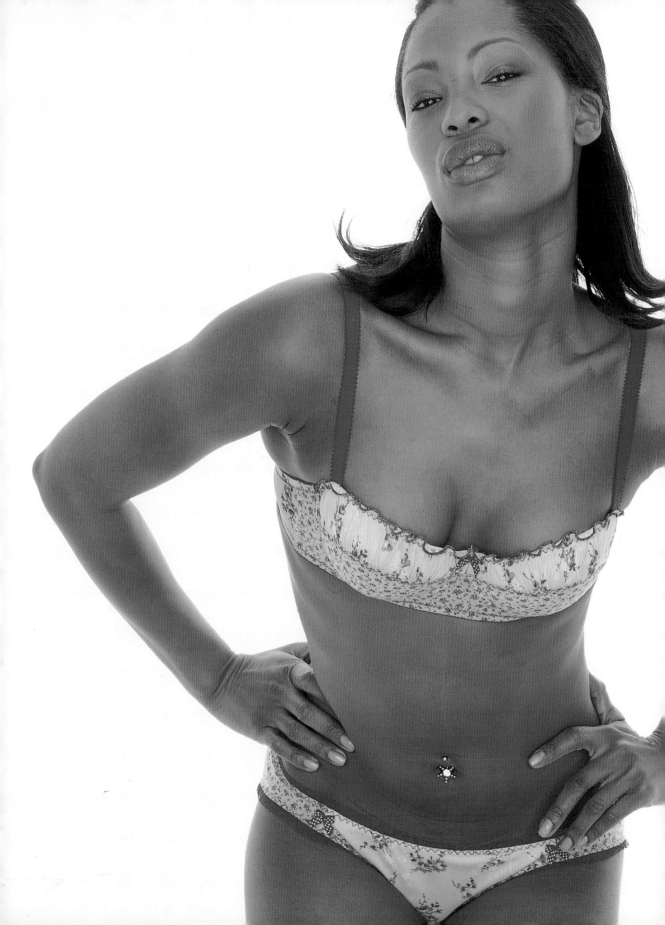

A woman's guide to sex

Kate Taylor

Photographs by Laura Knox

Illustrations by Kid Spaniard

FIREFLY BOOKS

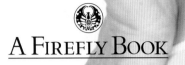

A FIREFLY BOOK

Published by Firefly Books Ltd. 2005

First printing

Publisher Cataloging-in-Publication Data (U.S.)
Taylor, Kate.
A woman's guide to sex / Kate Taylor ; photographs by Laura Knox ; illustrations by Kid Spaniard.
[256] p. : col. photos. ; cm.
Includes bibliographical references and index.
Summary: Advice for women on relationships, practicing sex and health matters.
ISBN 1-55407-097-X (pbk.)
1. Women — Sexual behavior — Popular works. 2. Sex instruction for women — Popular works.
3. Women — Health and hygiene — Popular works. I. Knox, Laura. II. Spaniard, Kid. III. Title.
306.7082 22   HQ29.T395 2005

Library and Archives Canada Cataloguing in Publication
Taylor, Kate, 1971-
A woman's guide to sex / Kate Taylor ; illustrator, Kid Spaniard ;
photographer, Laura Knox.
Includes index.
ISBN 1-55407-097-X
1. Sex instruction for women. 2. Women--Sexual behavior.
3. Interpersonal relations. I. Title.
HQ46.T39 2005   613.9'6'082   C2005-900107-0

Published in the United States by
Firefly Books (U.S.) Inc.
P.O. Box 1338, Ellicott Station
Buffalo, New York 14205

Published in Canada by
Firefly Books Ltd.
66 Leek Crescent
Richmond Hill, Ontario L4B 1H1

Editors: **Emma Dickens** and **Victoria Alers-Hankey**
Art director: **Simon Wilder** simon@shinydesign.demon.co.uk
Photographer: **Laura Knox**
Stylist: **Liz Hancock**
Illustrations: **Kid Spaniard**

Printed in Hong Kong

Contents

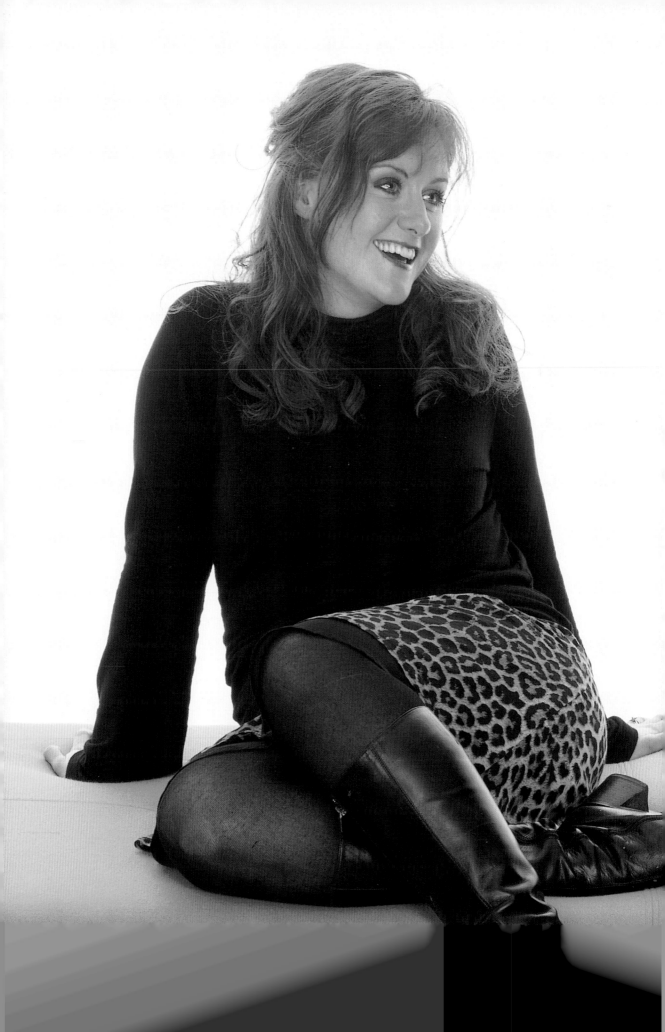

Introduction

Let's talk about sex. This book makes the most of women's greatest failing—the failing to be discreet about their sex lives. Unlike men (who usually morph into Trappist monks the moment sexual worries arise), women have the fabulous ability to spill their innermost secrets to anyone who'll listen.

Well, guess who was listening? Me. This book was inspired by the real-life sex lives of countless women. Over the years, as sex columnist for *GQ* magazine and as the presenter of the incredibly popular series *Sex Tips For Girls* and *More Sex Tips for Girls*, I received thousands of letters from women desperate to improve their partners' technique between the sheets. These fabulous women shared everything—their fears that their current blow-job technique was about as sexy as gargling with hotdogs, their insecurities and dilemmas, right through to the agonizing decision of when to sleep with a new man. The stories were always different but the premise was the same: women know they have the right to a fantastic sex life, but they don't know how to achieve it.

If that's you, I can assure you that the first steps to great sex are within this book. Whether you're an absolute beginner with nobody else to ask about what goes where, or a firebreathing goddess eager to brush up on advanced throat-lengthening skills—or even a mother who doesn't want the birth of her next baby to mark the death of her sex drive—you'll find tips in here to turn your sex life from fizzlin' to sizzlin'.

It's not just about the ins and outs of intercourse. For women, almost all sexual pleasure (or displeasure) begins way above the waistline. We're emotional creatures, and much of our libido is dictated by seemingly irrelevant factors like body image, emotional stability, even what we've had for dinner. So I've addressed these issues too—right up to sample menus for the ultimate first-date feast.

After reading *A Woman's Guide to Sex*, I'm hoping you'll be filled with confidence, armed with new ideas, and equipped with the skills to dazzle a new partner, or kick-start an old relationship. So while I'm dying for you to find that you can't put this book down, I wouldn't mind if your new sex life means you never get the time to pick it up. I want you to have amazing sex, sheet-scorching sex, tonight and every night for the rest of your life. And then I want you to tell me everything.

Kate Taylor

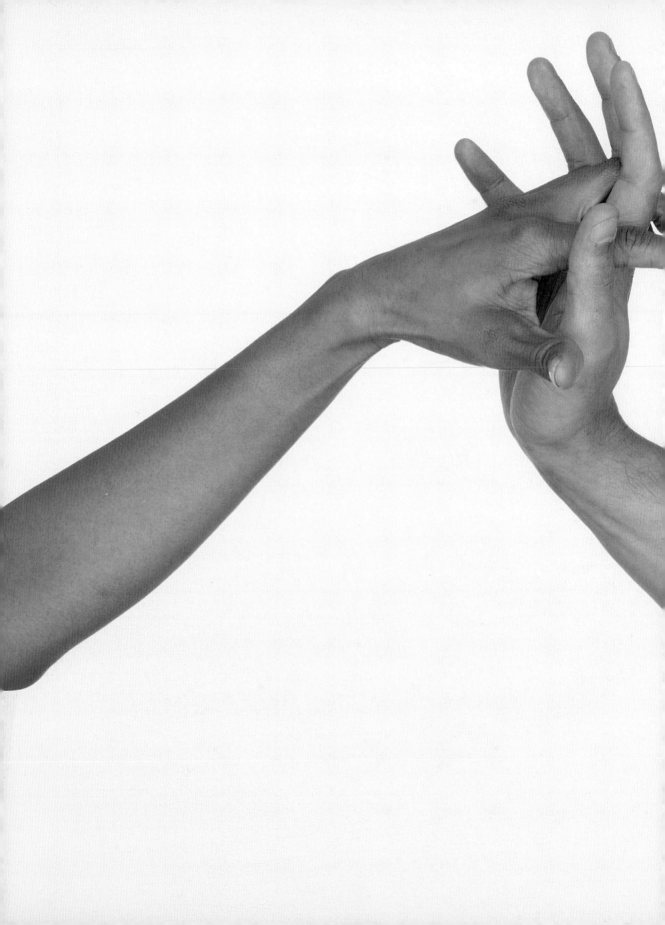

1 Are you good in bed?

So are you?

Ooh, that's the question, isn't it? It's what we all want to be. We want to be sexy and sexual, alluring and passionate. We want our current partner to be in a constant state of semi-lust, driven to distraction by thoughts of our naked body. We want our ex-lovers to be tortured by our memory, unable to enjoy sex with another woman because it's just not as great as it was with us. We want to be responsive, beautiful, bewitching and confident. We want to be good in bed.

So, are you? Well, you're going to be. Within these pages are the tips, techniques and tricks to make you very, very good in bed indeed. If you read the ideas here and include them in your sexual repertoire, you could easily be the best lover your partner (or future partners) has ever known. The reason is simple: most women don't bother to read sex books.

It's true. Most women you know won't ever have read a sex book. Instead, they go to bed with a head full of half-heard positions and some vague ideas about blow jobs, and just hope that the sex will be great. Unfortunately, women still believe in the White Knight theory of sex, that "When I meet the right man, the sex will be fantastic. He'll just *know* what my body needs to feel alive, and the simple touch of my hand on his hip will make him swoon with ecstasy." No, no, no. This is sweet but it's not true. It's like saying, "When I meet the right car, I'll just know how to drive." Really good sex

takes information and practice—lots of it. You have to know what goes where, why and how. Then you have to experiment like mad. Think of yourself as a nutty love professor, testing out new theories on your man—who'll be only too pleased to assist.

Your sexual appetite

Of course, it's easy to experiment in bed if you're happy to be there. To be great in bed you have to want to have sex. So, do you? The most likely answer is "sometimes." If you've met a new partner who you fancy like mad, you probably do. If you've been married for 30 years to a man who's losing his hair, teeth and mind, you may not. If you're going through menopause, you also might not. But if your period is due tomorrow, you probably do. So let's start here, with how you can boost your sexual appetite and get back your lust—for life.

Why work on your sexual appetite?

Before we begin, I have to have a quick word with anyone reading this who thinks that it's somehow wrong to be interested in having great sex, that it's somehow "dirty" or inelegant. Yes, I know we've all been sexually revolutionized but there are still women among us who have a "nice girls don't" mindset.

If this is you, please relax. It's fine to want sex. In fact, it's healthy, natural and good to

To be great in bed, you have to want to have sex. So do you?

want it. Sexual desire is an important, natural function in humans as it helps us reproduce—which is the single reason we're all on this Earth. Don't be afraid of your sexuality. Don't ever think it's wrong to want sex. No, no, sister! The only time that it's wrong is when you're using it for the wrong reasons—like, you think it'll make a man love you (it won't), or you think you'll be dumped if you don't sleep with him (in which case, don't you dare).

Sex at its best is shared between two people, in love, within a committed relationship. I am old-fashioned in that I don't believe women should sleep with men they don't care about. But that's not because I think they're sluts if they do; it's because I've seen them get hurt. Women bond when we have sex—hormones are released that physically cause our body to crave *his* body. You can't decide when that happens; there are some men that just get our bodies going crazy, so before we know it we are hopelessly in lust with someone we barely know (or only know bare).

By all means embrace your sexuality. Sex is a fabulous way to release tension, push the boundaries of your desires and explore your female essence. But be wise. Protect yourself. Don't sleep with any man until you know his true character. He is *entering* you, going deep inside you. Make sure you know who he is first. Anyway, back to your scheduled program …

Boosting your mojo

Do you feel sexy? If you do, you can skip ahead a few pages. In fact, we'll meet you at Chapter 2 for some killer tips on flirting. The rest of you, stick with me. There are many reasons why a woman can go from "Yes, yes, yes!" to "Dear God, no." The first ones I'll be dealing with are medical. We'll get these out of the way right now because if any of the following apply to you, you'll need specific help on boosting your love-vibe.

Menopause

As we mentioned before, menopause is a common time to lose your libido. Fluctuating hormone levels play havoc with your body, causing all kinds of things like hot flashes and headaches, which can make sex the last thing on your mind. However, you don't have to just put up with it and suffer. The repercussions of doing this could last long after your hot flashes have faded away. There are many treatments to consider so the best thing to do is look into what is available and consult your doctor or an alternative health practitioner.

If you don't like the idea of HRT, consider natural alternatives. Some women achieve great results from using natural hormone therapies, like progesterone creams rubbed directly into the skin. Other herbal supplements like evening primrose oil can also help.

Antidepressants

Some antidepressants—usually those classed as SSRI (selective serotonin reuptake inhibitor)—can inhibit arousal to the extent that you wouldn't get turned on even if Brad Pitt stood in front of you, butt-naked. They can also delay or even prevent orgasm. Again, consult your doctor. Some research has shown that Wellbutrin (aka bupropion HCl) has no such effects and can even boost your sexual appetite. More studies are needed, but in the meantime talk to those who know. Great sex is a natural mood enhancer, so, unless you are seriously depressed or in danger of harming yourself, it might be worth making the switch.

Drugs

Marijuana, cocaine, Ecstasy, speed and heroin can all affect sexual appetite. Yes, you can have what feels like great sex on all these drugs, but the aftereffects (shivers, paranoia, weepiness, depression) can leave your libido in tatters. So, say No to drugs and Yes to your man.

Prescribed drugs

Some prescribed drugs can ruin your lustiness. Sadly, they're saving your life at the same time. Common offenders are antiandrogen drugs, sedatives, cardiac drugs, ulcer medications and neuroleptics. Talk to your doctor if your sexual appetite (or responsiveness) has decreased after starting a drug. There may be alternatives.

Illness

Illness stops you feeling sexy. Not only does being unhealthy affect your sexual confidence, but your loss of libido is your body's way of saying, "Enough with the jiggy-jiggy! I'm trying to heal here." But if you have a long-term illness, you might not want to resign yourself to a lifetime of celibacy. Common causes of decreased lust are illnesses that raise prolactin levels (such as some pituitary conditions, hypothyroidism, cirrhosis and stress) and those affecting your ovaries and uterus (which can throw your hormone levels). Seek medical advice.

Other reasons

If there isn't a medical reason for you feeling about as up-for-it as a dead stick, the cause could be emotional. Sex is a personal issue, starting in our brains, and encountering stress, a big change or feeling unattractive can make the bedroom the last place you want to be (unless it's to curl up with a few candy bars to watch *Beaches*). The most common emotional reason for this is lack of sexual confidence. Reading this book should help, as having specific techniques to try out in bed will make you feel armed and ready. Read ahead and see if you start feeling more positive and aroused. If not, then come back here and establish whether it might be that you are suffering from more specific confidence issues.

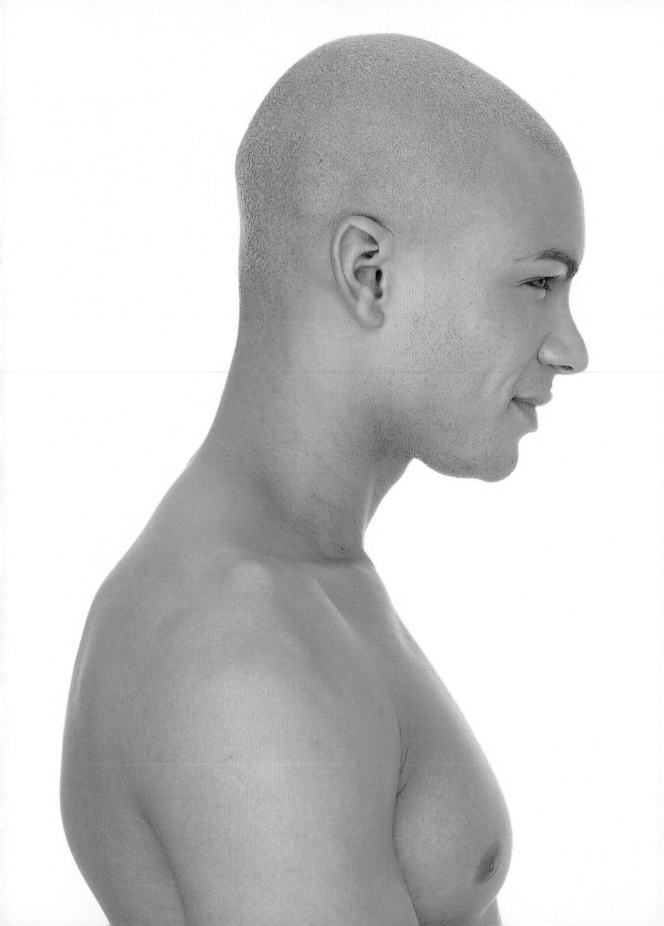

If you've noticed a lack of sexual confidence after you've met a new man, I suggest you take a good look at that relationship. Don't listen to what your friends and family think, listen to what you think. Those little voices in your brain are your instincts.

Lack of sexual confidence

Let's face it, which of us doesn't suffer from a lack of confidence in bed at one point or another? However, there comes a point where lack of sexual confidence starts impeding your pleasure. You'll know if you're there: negative thoughts about yourself and your sex appeal will crowd your brain all the time, not just when you're in bed. You'll begin to doubt your own opinions and tastes, you'll find it very hard to make decisions, and you might end up tearful, irrational and depressed.

But it doesn't have to be that way. If you suspect you might be even on the brink of losing your sexual confidence, I want you to take positive action immediately. Make a note of when you first noticed feeling this way. What had happened? Sometimes doubts can creep in when you're going through a big change (of job, lifestyle, home or partner) or when absolutely nothing has changed in your life for far too long. It is perhaps easiest of all to lose your oomph just by standing still.

Mr. Right or Mr. Wrong?

If you've noticed a lack of sexual confidence after you've met a new man, I suggest you take a good look at that relationship. Don't listen to what your friends and family think: listen to what *you* think. Those little voices that speak up in our brain are our instincts—ignore them at your peril. There might be little signs that he isn't Mr. Right after all. Does he criticize you or tease you constantly? Is he reliably unreliable? Do you feel that he should just be treating you better generally? Obviously don't set impossible standards for him—no, he shouldn't have proposed within two weeks of meeting you—but don't discount any shabby treatment either. Remember, men are at their most attentive at the beginning of a relationship. He won't warm up, so don't stick around waiting for Mr. Lukewarm to change into Mr. Motivated. It simply won't happen.

If you have nonnegotiables in your relationships that's a good thing. Believe in them. Be honest with yourself about what you want. If you are after a boyfriend who calls you every day, don't settle for one who always seems to have broken his dialing finger. If you want presents, ditch Mr. Thrifty and wait for Mr. Wallet. You will meet a man who fits your ideal perfectly (or so closely that it doesn't matter), but don't sell yourself short—believe in the process and keep looking.

What you should never, ever do is settle for an imperfect man who treats you badly because you don't believe you deserve better. You do. We all do. Somewhere out there is a man who will believe you hung the moon and the stars in the sky. I guarantee it. But ignoring your inner voice is the quickest way to end up depressed. (I know. Been there, dated him, swallowed the antidepressants.)

I'm not a yummy mummy

No matter what you actually look like after you've had a baby, you just will feel frumpy. It happens to every woman and it's a pain in the butt—even worse than the stitches. If you think this is you, read Chapter 7. Do not suffer in silence—there are quick fixes that can have you feeling fabulous again before your baby is even sleeping through the night.

I'm recently divorced

Eek—this is such a confidence destroyer. I've never been through it, but I can totally understand that there must be terrible feelings of inadequacy, failure and doom circling your brain like vultures in the desert. No wonder you don't feel like parading through the bedroom with somebody new.

Again, I urge you to break the pattern as soon as possible. It's so easy to sink into depression and end up there for years and years. The best that I can do is point you in the direction of a therapist (you can get referred through your doctor) and assure you that things will get better. Women are actually much more adept at coping with the end of relationships than men are—and more resilient than they think. Also, unmarried women are statistically half as likely to suffer from depression as married women. Remember that when you're seeing supposedly blissfully happy couples everywhere you look.

I've been raped or sexually abused

There are many organizations that are just waiting with open arms to help and support you. This isn't something you should ever try to cope with on your own. This was caused by somebody else. You didn't make it happen. Contact your local Rape Crisis Center or ask your doctor to recommend a suitable support group.

I'm in a rut

Are you? Is everything about you the same as it was five years ago? Do you look ahead and just see more of the same heading towards you with monotonous certainty? Then book a haircut and a manicure. I know, I know—but trust me. Ruts are notoriously comfy places. You have to light a fire under your butt to help you escape; a haircut is a tiny Bunsen burner. Somehow, changing your appearance in a nonpermanent way is the perfect motivator for changing other, scarier, parts of your life. It's impossible to be depressed with newly painted nails. Don't argue—just pick up the phone and make the appointment. Afterwards, other changes will occur to you. You might suddenly get an idea for changing the furniture in your living room, or an easy Internet business idea. Again, just do it. The idea here is to start liking yourself again. When you change, you get a sudden rush of pride. Even if it goes wrong, you'll feel better because you tried and put yourself on a mission. Believe me, it's true.

You will meet a man who is right for you—

so don't sell yourself short and settle for less.

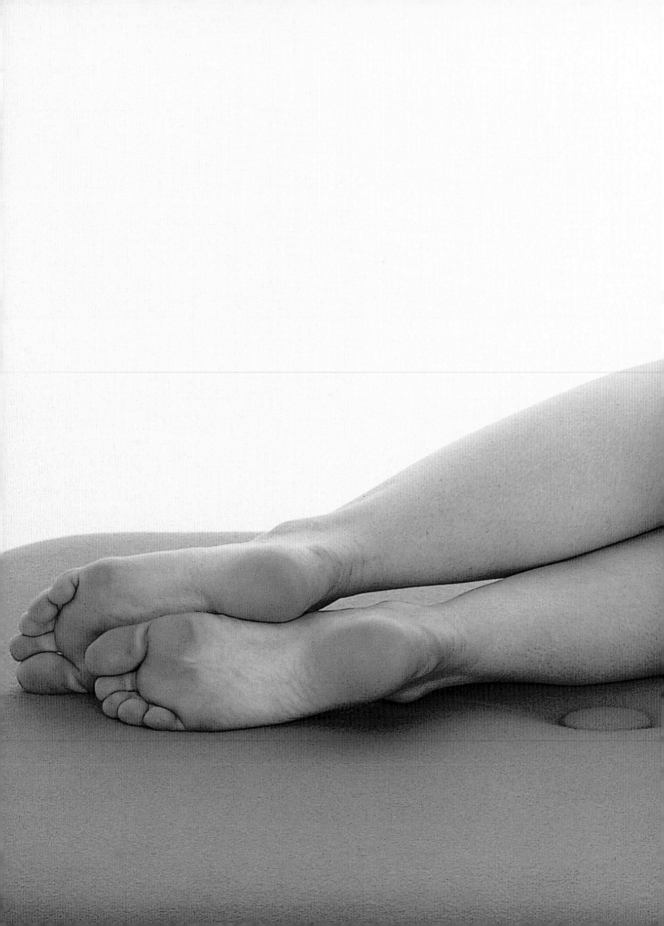

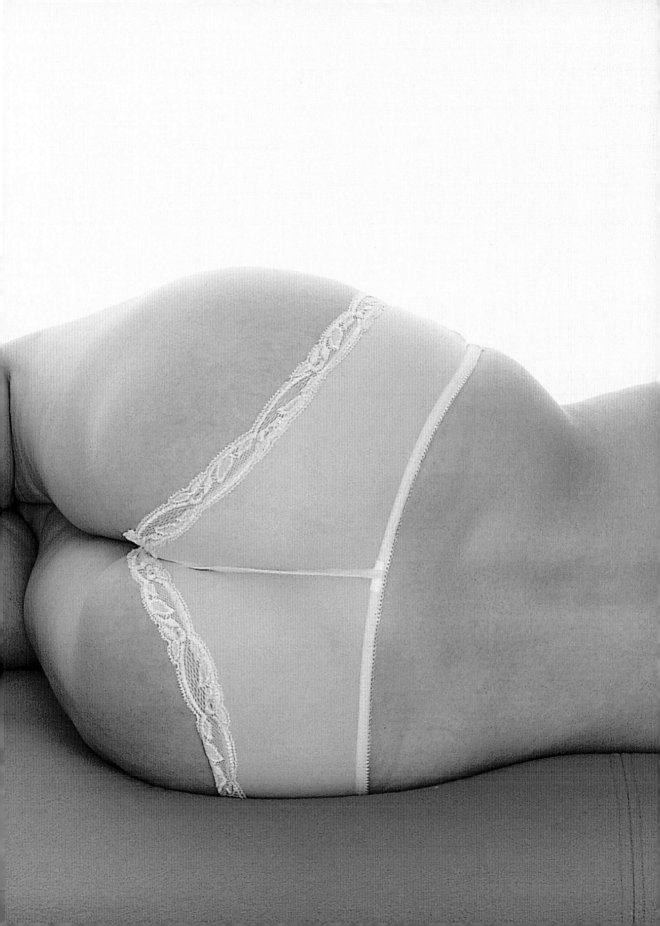

I married the wrong man

Maybe you did. Maybe your life would be way better if you'd never married him. Maybe by now you'd be sitting on a yacht married to a multimillionaire who loves you madly. Or, maybe you wouldn't. The thing is, you'll never know. So stop thinking of the might-have-beens and concentrate on the now-whats. You have three choices:

1. Stay and feel sorry for yourself.
2. Leave.
3. Stay and try to make it better.

Option 1) is nonsense. Option 2) is totally your choice and not to be rushed into (unless he is abusing you, in which case pack your bags). And Option 3) is worth a shot.

If you're criticizing your partner regularly, get a haircut. Again, changing your appearance is shifting your focus back on to you, which is where it needs to be if things are going to change. You can't change your man. No way, never, no. As an Italian grandmother would say, "Fahgeddaboudit." But you can change the way you react to your man. Are you nagging him? Do you not trust him to do anything in the house, in his career, raising your kids? Then you're probably exacerbating the problem by micromanaging him the whole time. The more you tell him what to do, the less he will do. Make a tiny vow that, for a week, you will answer any question of his with a simple,

"Whatever you think." You're not allowed to say anything else. Not another word. Just, "Whatever you think." (You could spice it up by adding the word "darling" at the end, but nothing else.)

Why? Because it will signal that you've stopped being the boss in the relationship. It will tell him, "I trust you to make the right decision." Yes, it's scary. Yes, it'll work. If you can do it for a week, you'll start seeing the man you married returning to you. Probably carrying flowers. Remember, the more you *respect* him, the more he will *cherish* you.

My body's weird

In her own words, here's Lily: "My left boob is bigger than my right one. It's been like that since they first started growing, when I was 13. Now it's about half a cup size bigger. I hate it. I get so embarrassed. I wear a chicken-fillet implant in my bra on the smaller side, so you don't notice anything when I'm dressed. But when I'm naked I think it really shows. It took me six months to be able to go bra-less in front of my boyfriend."

Here's Lily's boyfriend: "It's cute. This way I know it's her. Even in the dark."

Remember that scene in *Shirley Valentine* where she is being seduced by her Greek lover? He kisses her all over her stomach. She yells, "You kissed my stretch marks! Ewww!" He replies, "They are the marks of life." She was worried that her body didn't conform to the "norm," and he didn't give a damn.

When a man loves you, he loves you. He doesn't care about the "deformities" that are vast in your mind and teeny in his. In fact, he probably doesn't even notice them. He just wants to get horizontal. If you're in a loving, committed relationship, he honestly won't care about the little things that make your body different from another woman's. In fact, he'll rejoice in them. And if you're not in a loving, committed relationship, you shouldn't be doing it anyway. (There, I said it!) Never worry about your faults and flaws. All that others are aware of are their own. He's far too busy obsessing over whether you'll see that weird mole he has on the inside of his left buttock to pick on you.

And don't get hung up about your genitalia, either. Nobody's private parts are identical. We don't often get to see each others', but if you ever leaf through an adult magazine, you'll see the vast range of vaginas that Mother Nature has handed out. You'll see big labia, small labia, huge clitorises, tiny ones, red skin, pink, purple, gray … All are acceptable, all are beautiful, all deserve to be loved.

If you don't have medical issues, depression or a lack of sexual confidence but you still don't want to swing from the chandeliers, what's wrong with you? I think you probably just need to gear up your sensuality.

Increase your sensuality

Woman are sensual creatures. That means that we are tuned in to our senses, all five of them. Roughly speaking, this means that if things don't feel good to us, we don't feel good. Sadly, it's all too easy to let the sensual part of your life get neglected. You're busy, you're stressed, your life is hectic … Everything else seems like more of a priority. Before you know it, you're acting like a man—trying to fix all of your problems with logical solutions. While this sounds good in theory, it's not the answer. There's more to women than that. The reality is that it leaves your senses unfed and this usually results in a lack of libido.

So, you need to feed your senses again. Here's how to do it:

Boost your sense of touch

Book a massage
It'll relax you and help you to enjoy being touched again. Sometimes this is easier when it's a stranger who's touching us, in a totally nonsexual way. Relax and just concentrate on the sensation of another person's hands running over your skin.

Buy clothes that feel good
Tactile fabrics like velvet, fur (fake works just as well as real), satin, silk and cashmere all appeal

to our sense of touch. And of course they'll appeal to your man's. Try to wear something every day that is deliciously soft. If you can wear it next to your skin, it'll make you act like a cat—purring and languid. Always have nice bed linen and fabrics on your bed; invest in the most expensive cotton-rich sheets you can afford. Buy a warm, fur throw to snuggle under on colder nights. You'll be amazed how things that feel good make *you* feel good too.

Buy expensive underwear

Get your bra size properly measured if you haven't already, and splash out on the most expensive underwear you can afford. Wear it often. Most days if possible. And throw out the granny pants. Sexy underwear never fails to make you feel expensive and special, even if you're wearing it under track pants and a T-shirt and washing the car. Having such a simple, sexy secret with yourself makes a huge difference to your day—and if you have a partner it's obviously a great bonus for him too.

Take long hot baths

And then take time to smother yourself in body lotion all over. Scrub your skin with a loofah to slough off dead cells and make your body feel smooth as silk. Milk works well too—try adding a handful of powdered milk to the running water and just see how silky your skin feels by the time you emerge.

Boost your sense of smell

Use perfume every day

Don't save it for special occasions. Every day is a special occasion. If you can't afford fancy stuff, buy scented oils in yummy fragrances like vanilla or musk and add them to an unscented body lotion. Slather it on everywhere.

Light scented candles

Ylang-ylang is renowned for revving up your sex drive. Buy a set of scented tea lights (January sales are a good time for bargains) and use some at work, some by the bed and some by the bath. Heaven. Other good scents are sandalwood and cinnamon—men love them.

Stop smoking

Nothing will improve your sense of smell faster. After three days you'll be inhaling the air like a mad mountain climber.

Nuke nasty odors

The best, cheapest way to freshen your space is to fill a spray bottle with a mixture of half water, half fabric softener. Spray everywhere and leave to dry. Miraculous.

Guarantee intimate freshness

Drinking a glass of unsweetened cranberry juice every day keeps your more, um, southerly regions smelling fresh as a daisy. Speaking of which …

Buy yourself flowers

Don't wait for the man in your life to step up to the florists. Instead, buy your own. Indulge yourself with the biggest bouquet you can afford, as often as you can afford it. If you think it's an extortionate waste of money, buy houseplants like orchids that will thrive inside and scent your room.

Boost your sense of taste

Eat good, natural food

This is such an easy habit to acquire and once you've tasted delicious, freshly squeezed pomegranate juice, or bitten into giant chunks of sweet cantaloupe melon, you'll be a sensual-food addict. Buy the best you can afford. Fresh-ground coffee, newly baked bread, lavender honey, thick sweet cream … This is sexy stuff. Don't save it for the bedroom—make every meal a sensual experience. Eat off nice plates (junk shops are great for picking up beautiful bargains) and use soft, white linen napkins.

Eat smaller meals

Everything tastes better when you're hungry. Do as the Japanese do and practice "Hari Hachi Bu." This roughly translates as: "Eat until you are 80 percent full." In Japan, the Okinawa people follow this principle through their lives and live until they're over 100.

Musturbation

I made that word up. Like it? I was trying to think of a way to express that masturbating is a fun, healthy, sexy thing that every woman can—and should—do. Before we get into the ins and outs of sex with the big boys, you should take some time out to explore your sex drive on your own.

Why you should masturbate

Just for a moment, let's separate sex and sexuality. Sex is something that you do with someone else. But your sexuality is yours alone. It's your own body's interest and appetite for all things sexual. You're never going to know your sexuality properly until you discover it solo. You won't find the magic switch with somebody else—there's too much else going on. They'll put you off your stride, you'll confuse them. Not good. Instead, own your sex drive by stimulating it by yourself.

There's absolutely no need to get hung up about masturbation. Think how unapologetic men are about it—boastful even. Why should they have all the fun? It's in no way dirty or wrong—and thankfully the taboo that surrounds it is beginning to be lifted. It doesn't mean you are weird, or desperate, or that you can't and never will find a man to have sex with. It doesn't mean you're a sex-starved slut who lives only for pleasure. You won't go blind and you won't grow hairy palms.

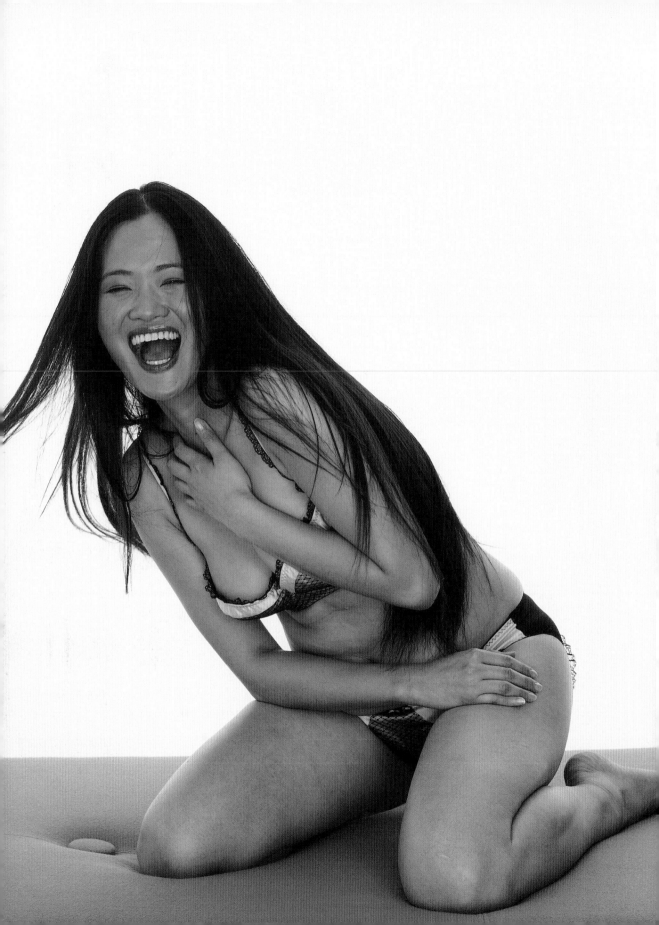

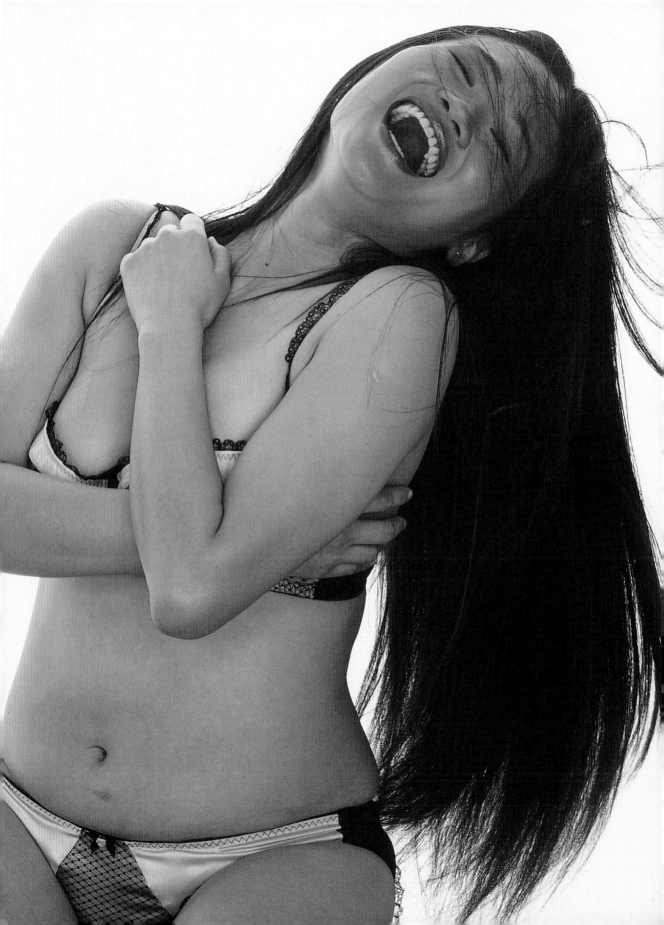

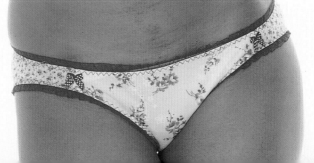

Good underwear makes you feel expensive and special.

Having this secret will make a huge difference to your day.

How to masturbate

Find a place where you won't be disturbed. Turn the phone off, and close the curtains. It is best not to be disturbed. Yes, there is a time and a place to be "caught" masturbating, but it's much later, when you're in a long-term relationship and you've forgotten his birthday. If you can, dress your bed with some fabrics like fake fur or silk sheets. Light a scented candle. Turn the lights down low and the heat up. Gather together some props to help you. Good things include:

● Lubrication (K-Y Jelly, AstroGlide, baby oil).
● Something to read (men's magazines like *Fiesta* or *Forum* have some interesting articles. Or you could read a collection of sexual fantasies, like Nancy Friday's *My Secret Garden*. Otherwise, some softcore erotica like the Black Lace series for women are a good bet).
● A vibrator.
● A mirror (some women enjoy watching themselves masturbate).

Start by massaging your breasts, paying attention to how they respond to your touch. See how your nipples harden as you become aroused. Feel the soft skin under your hands, and note how good they must feel to your lover. (Don't telephone him to tell him that. Keep your mind on your work, missy.)

Thinking rude thoughts, run your hands down to your panties, stroking your inner thighs and teasing yourself by slipping a finger just under the material. Let your mind wander along with your hands. Everything is allowed.

Now, using lubricant, explore your vagina with your fingers. Hold the lips open with one hand and start gently stimulating your clitoris with the other. You might prefer rubbing one side of the clitoris, or placing a finger on either side and rubbing in circular motions. You might like to tap it with a fingertip.

If you've got a vibrator, turn it to the lowest speed and run it all over your vaginal area, slipping it inside you and then rubbing your clitoris. See if you can find your G-spot, by angling the tip up toward your tummy. If you feel an area that's extra-sensitive, concentrate your efforts there for a moment.

There are more specific tips in Chapter 6, but don't get hung up on technique right now. This is all about pleasing yourself and letting your hands and mind wander. What feels good? Do you like direct clitoral stimulation with no buildup at all? Or do you prefer being teased before your vagina is touched? Do you like stroking your butt while you do it?

Concentrate on what thoughts arouse you, too. In fact, gather as much information as you can about what turns you on and how you like to be touched. Without this, you'll never fully know your own sexuality.

Here's how some women like to masturbate:

Susy, 23: I love to have my nipples pinched, but don't have enough hands to do it all, so I use clothespins.

Katy, 38: I place the tip of my middle finger on the tip of my clit, then my index and ring fingers either side of it. Then I press them against the base my clit over and over again. It's simple but the feeling is amazing.

Fiona, 45: I love to masturbate with an ice cube inside my vagina. No words can express what the chill inside feels like.

Katherine, 50: Direct clitoral stimulation works best for me. I wet my fingers from my mouth, or between my legs, or with K-Y. Then I use the first two fingers of both hands to spread the skin a little, the others to stroke. It's fabulous to begin stroking the center of the clitoris, then while continuing the strokes, move them around, then down, now and then bringing them stroking back into the center. It's a self-tease and the resulting orgasm is wonderfully intense. Watching with a mirror makes it even better.

Helen, 33: I take a wet, warm facecloth and put Vaseline on it. Then I stroke it up and down over my clit. I tease myself for as long as I can, then press it hard against my vagina.

Jules, 22: I lie on my bed with my legs in the air and spread wide. Usually, I prop them against the headboard. I rub my clit gently in a circular motion, getting more and more intense as I get more and more horny. When I get really aroused, I use my legs to thrust my lower torso into the air, up and off of the mattress.

Maria, 43: I like to rub a dildo against my clit with a massaging motion. Then I tease myself by putting the head of the dildo inside me then taking it out and rubbing it against my clit again. I do this until it just drives me crazy, until I put the whole dildo inside me.

Sasha, 29: When no one is home, I stack several pillows on top of each other. I lay a towel over the top one—the terrycloth is an amazing stimulator. Mount the pillows and rub back and forth. You almost don't even slide, it's more of a rocking motion. As I get to the end, before I climax, I stop, play with my nipples a while, and start again. I do this a few times. It takes time, but it's worth it in the end, trust me. When I finish my last "round" I put a small stuffed toy under the top pillow, so I have something a little firmer to ride. Use anything you like. Or just use the pillows. It's up to you. The orgasm is intense and amazing.

Off you go, then, and we'll see you in Chapter 2. Have fun ...

Q+A

■ My boyfriend isn't interested in sex. When I question him he says it feels like a very "animal" thing. I try to make advances but he pushes me away. Is there anything I can do?

● The best thing you can do when a man goes off sex is to try and go off it too. I know that sounds crazy but bear with me. If you keep making advances, it's likely to push him even farther away from the whole idea. If the sex was fine in the beginning, something must have happened to quell his passion. I'd guess that he was stressed about something (stress is men's number-one passion killer) except that he said sex feels like "a kind of animal thing." That suggests that it's an emotional problem. Are you being romantic toward him? Could he possibly feel that sex is all you want from him? Men get weird when they feel they're being "used" for sex. Basically, men like to be the sexual hunters, and they expect us to provide all the mushy business. Stop being the sexual hunter —i.e., stop making any advances sexually for a while—and the chances are he'll relax. He'll feel the pressure is off him to perform. Then, if you step up the romance a little (call him a bit more often, be more reassuring) he'll know you want more than his body. Which is about when he'll start giving you his body again. Good luck.

■ My sister-in-law advised me to put off sex for as long as is humanly possible when I first meet a man. Does this really keep a guy interested? I thought we weren't supposed to play games.

● Women who say "we're not supposed to play games" are always single. And it's always us married types who dole out old-fashioned advice like *don't do it with him*. That's got to tell you something, hasn't it? Your sister-in-law is right—putting off sex is a great idea. Yes, it keeps a man interested in you, incredibly so. If you've never done it, it's worth trying—the rewards are huge. But there are benefits aside from having a man truly fall in love with you: you'll feel better. When we have sex, we release a bonding hormone called oxytocin which drives us nuts: we obsess over the man, think about him constantly, pursue him relentlessly and put up with anything to get another "fix." It's not our fault; it's chemical. But oxytocin doesn't get released if you don't have sex. Next time, put off sex for as long as you possibly can—at least three months, but ideally six. The rewards will speak for themselves. And don't think of it as playing games. Think about it as guarding your heart. I'm telling you, the joy of having a man really love you, getting married and building a family is far more intense than the joy of sex.

■ I'm involved with a man who I don't think is very good for me. We're opposite in every way possible. I would just finish with him but the sex is the best I've ever had. When we're together, I feel that he is the best man in the world for me. But when we're apart, all the reasons against seeing him come back into my brain. I'm lost and confused.

● You, my darling, have fallen in lust. This is so incredibly common that I'd wager almost half of all couples are together because of their strong sexual attraction. Is that so wrong? Well, yes, if it's all you've got in common. But no, if you share other stuff too, good stuff, like a sense of humour, basic moral values and a few interests. The thing to do is take a break from him. Just for a couple of weeks. Get some space and make a decision when your hormones aren't raging. Make a list of how you feel when you're away from him and how you feel when you're together. Does he make you happy? Does he make you laugh? If you feel safe, warm and secure when you're together, I'd say that you could do all right with him. But if he makes you feel insecure and uncomfortable, buy yourself a vibrator and ditch the guy. Lust is fine when it's accompanied by companionship and fun, but it's not enough on its own. Good luck.

■ I'm 34, and after several years of short-term relationships and flings, I'm beginning to think I'm incapable of anything long term. The many men I meet are attentive and enthusiastic initially, and then they stop trying and I get fed up. Am I too demanding? Or a commitment-phobe?

● You're not too demanding and I doubt you're a commitment-phobe. What you're describing is the "three-month itch," when a guy changes from an eager beaver into a sloth. This happens when he feels comfortable and secure, and when he relaxes after the pursuit. He is saying, "I've done my work. Now, what are you going to do for me?" It's incredibly irritating. With the next guy take things slower. He won't keep chasing unless you keep running away. Don't sleep with him so soon. Don't call him. Don't suggest dates. In short, be more elusive. He'll be so caught up in the thrill of the chase that the three-month mark will whizz by without him realizing. Modern girls feel it's only fair to do half the work in a relationship, but it doesn't work that way. Men are happiest when they're providing for us, making us happy and dreaming up exciting dates to take us on. If you don't recognize that, it's because you're not allowing men to treat you right. Be more of a challenge —your relationships will last a lot longer.

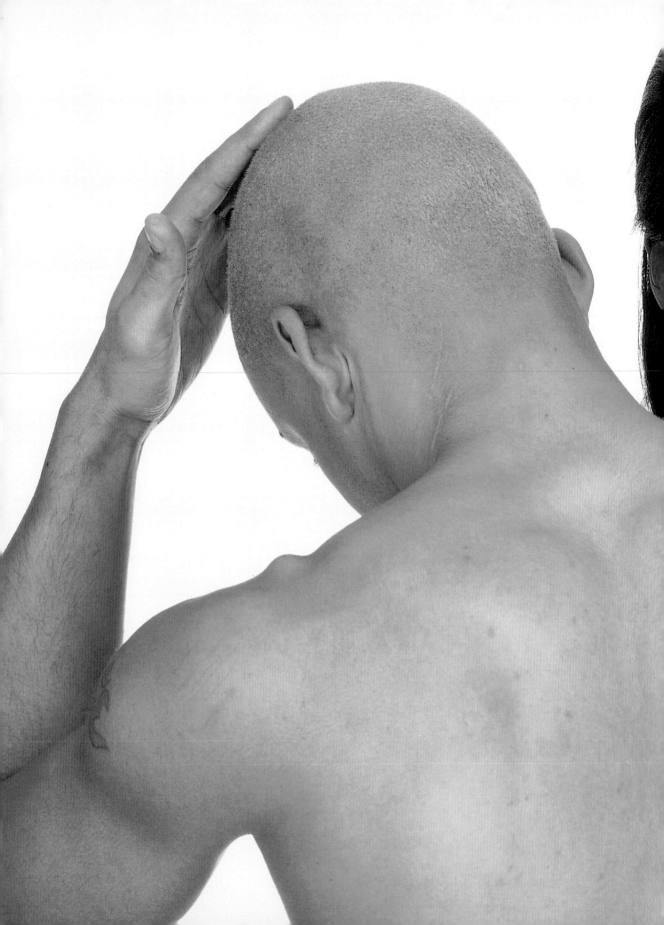

2 Flirtysomething

(develop your powers of attraction)

Personal story: **How to be a woman**

I'm a reformed non-flirt. When I was younger, in my late teens and twenties, I'd never bother to flirt with men. I'm part of that generation of women who believed we had to make our way in a man's world by being like men. My mother is a housewife and she was always telling me not to make the same mistakes she made, and to concentrate on getting a good career. At university I was quite plain and my clothes were "thrift-store chic." I had loads of male friends. They'd stay in my room until all hours chatting (usually about the girls they liked) and I prided myself on being able to talk to them like a guy.

I had girlfriends who thought the way I did—we dissed "girly girls," and spent hours pondering why all the men chased after them, when they could have had smart, intelligent women like us. We didn't get it. Why were men falling over themselves to date girls who wore ribbons in their hair and couldn't talk about anything more interesting than getting a manicure?

After college I landed a great job at a men's magazine and it was more of the same. The men liked talking to me because I was smart and guy-ish, but they lusted after the models. Have you ever met a model? In real life? They drifted into the office, usually late, and just sat there while the art department looked through their portfolios. If they'd got lost on the way in they almost boasted about it. They were scatterbrained, smiley and—here's that word again—girly.

It was the same situation: men talked to me all night, but it was models they wanted to date. I didn't get taken out for dinners or to parties. I was invited to after-hours drinks with a gang of guys. They pinched my cigarettes but never my ass. I was one of them. A guy.

It took me 10 more years to figure out that maybe, just maybe, men preferred talking to women who weren't masculine. I joined an Internet chat room where women discussed the ploys they'd used to attract men. It was a revelation—there were acres of words all about being feminine. One women ran a whole discussion group about hair. Just hair. How to style it, look after it, and how to grow it long. "Why long?" I wrote, fingering my chic chin-level hair nervously. "Because the men like it long," she replied. "Long hair is feminine. Men don't want women who act or look like men."

I'm quite proud of myself that I was adaptable enough to change. I started slowly—instead of dominating the conversation on dates, I let him do most of the talking. I let him make the jokes. I really thought they'd think of me as brainless and stupid, but I was wrong. They loved it! They thought nothing about me; they thought all about themselves. The smarter I made them feel, the more they liked me.

I girlied-up my apartment. Out went the framed quotes from Gloria Steinem; in came fluffy cushions and pink lampshades. I went through a brief phase of having everything leopardskin, and I've never been so popular with guys. I grew my hair long, I got regular manicures, I relegated my thick jeans and Timberland boots to the back of the wardrobe.

I also got used to being perverse, unpredictable, capricious. Before, I'd always tried to reason with men, thinking they'd appreciate my ability to think logically. They didn't. Instead, I started having fun. If they invited me out on a masculine date (like greyhound racing), I complained that my heels would sink into the mud by the track. Did they laugh scornfully? No! They offered to carry me. They paid for dinner. They started boasting about how strong they were (they had to be, to carry *me*) and they started remembering my birthday.

The more womanly I became, the more romantic men became. I got flowers, Valentine's cards, taken home to meet mothers. I got picked up and dropped off. I got treated like a woman. Never was I accused of being unreasonable or stupid (the two things I'd dreaded). Instead, men fell over themselves to solve my problems, to fix my stuff, to slay my dragons. And to marry me. I got three proposals in two years.

I wouldn't ever switch back. I've modified my girliness since those days (the pink lampshades have gone), but I've kept the basic principal. Men like feminine women. Now I never offer men advice, I don't listen to dating problems anymore, and I never even offer to pay my own way. I don't send Valentine's cards and I don't try to impress men—I let them impress me. It works. I get treated like a queen, like a model, like a woman.

Liz, 33

Why you should be a flirt

Flirting is feminine. It comes from your feminine energy. At its simplest, flirting is making other people feel good about themselves. That's very feminine—nurturing, caring. Women excel at this. So, you should be a flirt, and flirt at every opportunity, because it will help you tap into your feminine energy, which will mean you have more fun in your life and more successful relationships.

That sounds deep. I'm going to lighten up, because that's Rule 1 of successful flirting:

Kate's law of flirting

1. Be lighthearted

If you're terrified of flirting (and who isn't, especially with men they like), it might help to hear that good flirting is all very lighthearted. In fact it's all just words, so you don't have to panic about draping your hand casually over a man's thigh during conversation, or whatever. I think of it as SASS: Sugar Added to Social Situations, and it's just making a man feel good about himself.

Keep it light

Don't get drawn into serious conversations when you first meet a man. Don't try to dazzle him with your brain, and don't try to solve the world's problems. This is tough for most of us— modern women tend to think we should impress men with our brains rather than our beauty—

but it is important. Men prefer women who are "sexy diversions". This was true in the 1800s and it's still true today. If you are serious in your nature, he will come to associate you with serious issues. He will feel you need to be taken seriously, and will worry about what to talk to you about. And he might eventually decide not to bother.

Instead, keep those initial conversations on a light level. Yes, you can tease him. You can express your ideas, but don't get sucked into a conversation about heavy things, no matter how fascinating you find them. By "heavy," I mean any subject where your tone will change from casual banter into earnest discussion or, worst of all, preaching. This isn't about dumbing down. It's about lightening up. Flirting is not about being serious. There is a time and a place for everything. From you he should receive warmth and laughter.

Laugh at his jokes

And include him in your conversations. Remember things he told you and ask about them next time. Be *nice*. If he phones, sound pleased to hear from him (he'll phone more). Use lighthearted names for him like "hand-some" or "gorgeous." If he obviously considers himself wiser than Ghandi, go one step further and tell him he's wiser than God. But keep it light: only respond to the here-and-now. Don't do heavy stuff like seek him out and tell him

Flirting isn't about dumbing down. It's about lightening up. It's not about being serious. There is a time and a place for everything and this is the time that he should receive warmth and laughter from you.

You should be a flirt, and flirt at every opportunity, because

that you've been up all night thinking about something he said—that's way too much. At the time tell him he's fascinating, pile it on thick, then leave it at that.

I know what you're thinking: "Won't he think I'm in love with him if I start doing all that?"

No! That's the beauty—it's all just words. Men realize (unlike women) that words are just fluff and nonsense; it's actions that really count. Which is why the second Rule is:

2. Your words are keen but your actions are cool

If you can master this, you will be queen of all you survey. This is the true technique of flirting: it makes you enchanting, mysterious and unlike other girls. Because even while you're telling him that he is truly the most handsome, clever man you've ever met, you're putting your coat on to leave. Keep your actions the opposite of your words. Your words are a tropical rainforest, hot and heady; but your actions are Greenland.

You do this naturally with men you're not interested in. Imagine this—you're on a sort-of date with a man you aren't too keen on. On the way home he tells you that he doesn't think you should be getting too excited, he'd still like to see other women for a while, until he knows you better. Obviously you're astounded by his nerve. You make a silent vow right then and there not to give this Lothario another speck of your time. You don't e-mail him about it, or try to discuss it, you just make a mental note: "Loser." And that's it. You never see him again.

However, the same thing happens with a man you're secretly nuts over. He says the exact same words. Do you react identically? If you do, you're fabulous. But if, like the rest of us, you don't, you're in trouble. "Hmmm," you think. "Well, okay. This is actually quite grown up. I mean, it's very mature not to get involved too soon. After all, I might meet someone else tomorrow. This is a good idea." So you agree, and next time he calls, you go out with him.

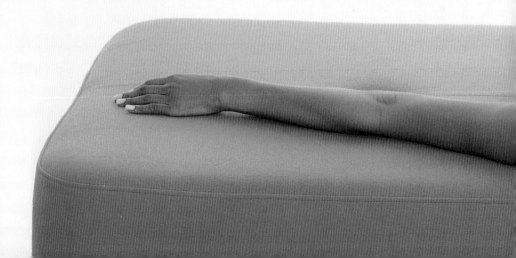

it will　help you tap into your feminine energy.

Now he knows you're keen. Your actions (seeing him again) prove that you will accept bad treatment from him, so guess what? That's what he'll give you from now on.

All men test us sometimes. They call up at the last minute saying things like, "I know we said we'd go out to dinner tonight, but I'm really tired. How about you come over and cook for me instead?" Should you agree? No. It's not a real question; it's a test. He's really saying, "I'm spending a lot of money on you, and doing a lot of stuff, and it's starting to add up. I'd like to know if I still need to do these things to keep you. Will you still love me if I treat you lazily?"

The answer should always be, "No."

3. Be the bearer of good news

This is how to be charming. Always pass on nice things you've heard about someone. Always. But never pass on bad stuff. If someone is being malicious about them, they're not going to hear it from you. Make it your vow.

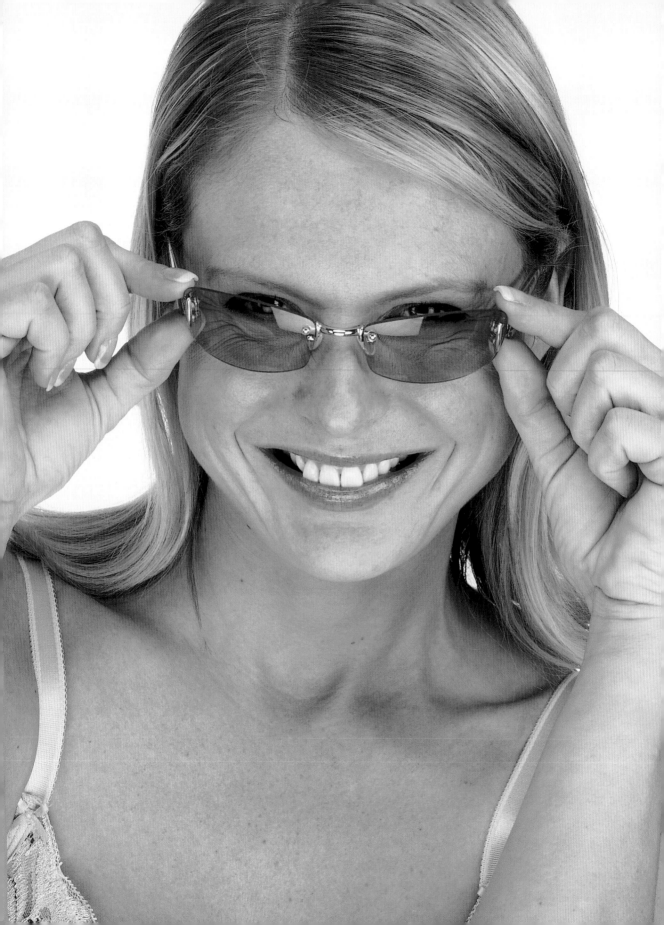

Similarly, pass on good news about yourself. When someone asks how you are, you're "Fabulous." When they ask why you've never been married, reply, "Because I said no." People like happy people who are doing fun things with their lives. Be the fun person who's always cheerful. If you want to confess your miseries, book a therapist.

4. Flirt with everyone

That means men and women. No, you won't suddenly have hoards of gay women asking you for dates. It's just that true flirts, true charmers, don't save their niceties for people they find attractive. They flirt with everyone—old ladies, sales clerks, waiters, their boss, their parents.

Why? Well, true flirts do it unconsciously. If you need a reason, think of it as covering your bases. If you flirt with a man, he will know you like him. If you flirt with a man and all his friends, he will know you're flirtatious. You won't have lost any of your mystery, he'll still get that itching sensation that he can't quite work you out, which he loves.

It's also good practice. Remember, flirting is just SASS. It's not sprawling on your desk with your skirt over your head. Just be as charming as possible to everyone you meet—even nasty people. Everyone responds to it and it's the fastest way to boost your social life and start meeting more men.

5. Accept every invitation to meet people

Dates don't count—this refers to parties, book launches, shopping evenings, yoga classes … Whenever somebody asks you to an event where you will be surrounded by lots of other people, accept their invitation. Without enough stimulation, your "social gene" will shrivel up and die. The only way you're going to learn to be good at flirting, speaking and meeting new people, is to practice.

How can I meet more men?

The only way is to go out more, and practice being approachable. If you are constantly out of the house but you never get chatted up, I'd guess that your body language is putting men off. So, try some of these tips:

1. Don't hunt in packs

If you're always in big groups of women, you won't get chatted up by anyone nice. It would take a very overconfident man to attempt to break into a large group, which explains why only lecherous drunks approach you in clubs. Whenever you can, break away from the group. Go to the bar alone, stand by the dance floor for a while, alone, walk about by yourself. Single yourself out—break away from the pack like a young gazelle, and you'll get attacked by lions. (And that's a good thing.) Better still, visit coffee shops and restaurants on your own.

Several women I know met their husbands this way. No, you won't look like a loser with no friends. A man who likes the look of you won't even think like that. He'll just be wondering how to talk to you. You, the mysterious enchantress at the table for one.

2. Carry a conversation-starter

Read a book with a provocative title, something men can comment on. (Something unrelated to relationships, of course—not, *How To Get Any Man To Marry You Within 30 Days*.) Wear a pin or button with tiny writing on it, and watch people, strangers, driven to distraction as they try to read what it says. You'll get people crossing the room because they just have to know. (Try it and see if I'm wrong.) You can have pins made up in jewelry shops. Wearing a T-shirt with a message emblazoned across the front can work as well, but is slightly less classy and can be read from farther away, so men don't have to talk to you while they're reading.

When you go to a party, always carry an unusual handbag, or wear a bizarre bracelet, or a zany dress, your craziest shoes or tantilizing eye makeup. Always. At a party you have to be the one that stands out in a crowd. But only wear or do one of these things. Crazy shoes worn with zany dress, bizarre bracelet and unusual shoes doesn't say "alluring," it says, "My apartment was on fire and these were the only clothes I could rescue."

3. Advertise

Or, as my gay best friend calls it, "tits and teeth." Smile a lot, and expose one body part. (Only one.) Choose from cleavage, legs, or back. Okay, I'll give you shoulders and arms, too. The combination of a winning smile (it makes you look happy, which attracts) paired with a flash of flesh usually breaks down most male defenses like a wrecking ball.

4. Don't wear any rings on your left hand

Men do look to see if you're wearing a sparkler on your ring finger. Don't confuse the poor things by wearing rings all over your left hand so they have to burst their eyeballs to see. (Or don't do the other, hideous, thing of wearing a ring on every finger *except* your wedding finger—too tacky.) Make life easy for males: keep your left hand bare.

5. Show your waist

This is a psychological thing. Men are attracted, biologically, to women with narrow waists in comparison to hips. There's a specific term: the waist/hip ratio. It goes right back to caveman days, because women with a narrow waist/wide hips combo are more likely to conceive. It's why men go crazy for hourglass figures like Marilyn Monroe's. Worried your waist is too wide? Fake it, by wearing skinny-fit tops with baggier pants. Those cut with pockets on the hips will help add a few inches. Or just expose that sexy curve where your waist flares out just above your hip-bone—wear low-slung jeans and a small T-shirt.

Don't smother your shape. Choose coats that are cut to form a waist. If dresses don't fit enough at the waist, have them taken in. Buy suits with fitted jackets. I'm serious—this is powerful stuff. If the fashion is straight-up-and-down, mix the two. Buy some cheaper straight-cut outfits to look modern, but invest your money in classics cut with a softly defined waist. Always keep coming back to the classic looks that last. Men will always love women with waists. It's in their nature.

How to be sexy

You should try and be sexy every day, wherever you are. But what is sexy? Some women think that sexiness is talking about sex—referring to their sex lives, telling rude jokes or forwarding dirty emails. Is this sexy? No. That's acting like a guy, again, which (by definition) is not going to be sexy to other guys. Sexiness is acting like a woman. Sexy is …

1. Being clean and organized in your daily life

Clean, organized women look like their life is in order. This is sexy because it shows a man that you take care of yourself. You have high self-esteem. You're not a woman who needs rescuing, who is going to fall into his life and require 24/7 management. So clean out your handbags, get your shoes reheeled when they need it, wear clean clothes and keep a clean house. The exception to this rule is your hair and dress—occasionally you can be disheveled, with rumpled hair and slightly askew clothing (as long as it's all clean). In contrast to your usually immaculate dress, this will give a man the idea of how you look after you've just had riotous mad sex. (Yes, men are this basic.)

2. Looking healthy

This really means "looking fertile." Men are attracted to fertile women. So most beauty tips actually make you look healthier—shiny, thick hair, clean white teeth, wide-open eyes, rosy cheeks and a slim, strong figure are signs of health. And a healthy woman is a fertile woman. Never subscribe to that white-faced Dracula look. In real life, it repels men. You want to look like you can do it all night and still be bright and breezy in the morning.

3. Looking composed

"Composed" is a funny, old-fashioned word for "having your shit together." It means you never look anxious (so unsexy), insecure, unprepared or nervous. The easiest way to achieve composure is to shut up. Nervous people babble. Think "serene"—if you're nervous, close your mouth and smile. Sit still, no fidgeting. Breathe slowly. Make your

Make your actions confident, slow everything down: even your walk.

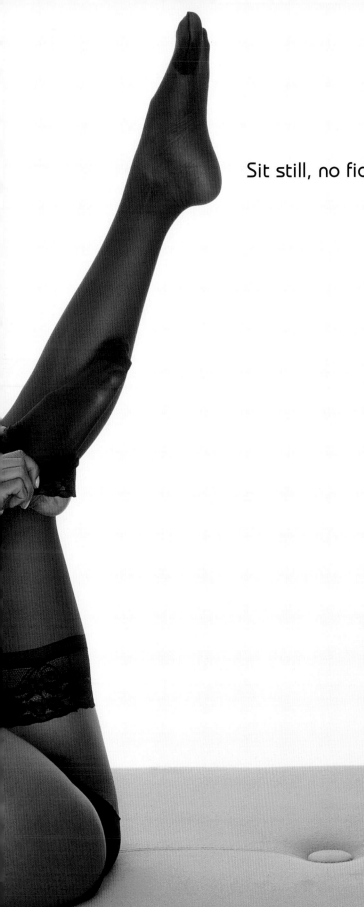

Sit still, no fidgeting. Even breathe slowly.

Looking healthy is one of the best hints I can give you. Most beauty tips actually make you look healthier—shiny, thick hair, clean white teeth, wide-open eyes, rosy cheeks and a slim, strong figure. A healthy woman is a fertile woman.

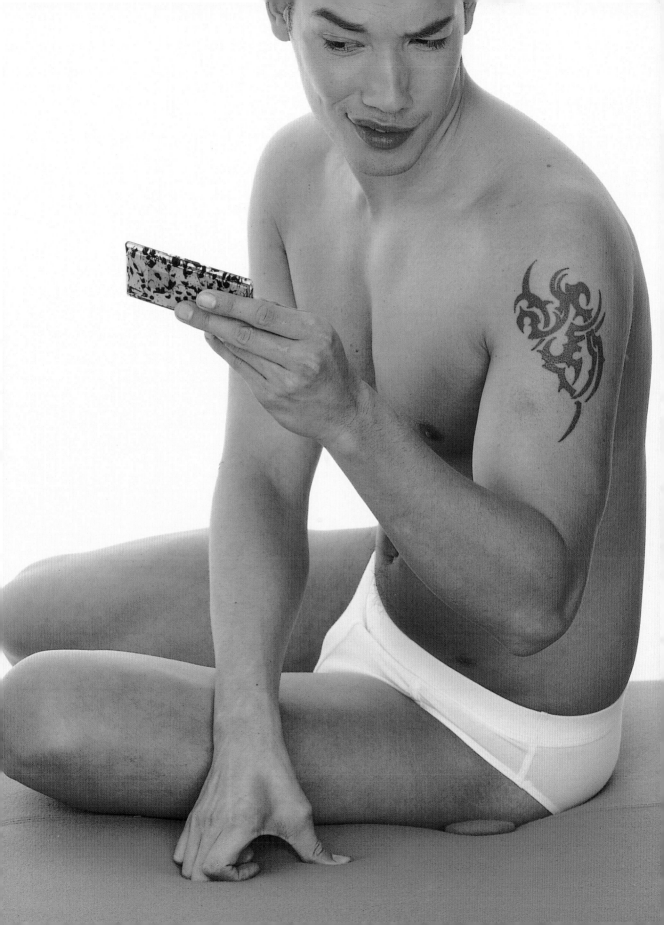

actions those of a confident woman. Slow everything down: even your walk. This gives the impression of being together. (Which means the boys can't wait to get into your life and mess it up again.)

Don't let men catch you off-guard. If you're on a date and he asks you something that you don't want to tell him (like why your last relationship ended, or why you've never been married, or why there's a security tag on your leg and an armed guard outside your apartment), you don't have to answer. You really don't. He's not a quizmaster; you won't lose points if you pass. Take a deep breath, smile and reply, "Why do you ask?" The only answer he can truthfully give is "because I'm nosy", so he won't. The pressure is now back on him and he'll retreat from this line of questioning, and that little incident with the police and the restraining order will remain unexplored.

If a man that you're still getting to know asks you on a date to do something that you don't want to, never be scared to refuse and turn him down. Trust that he wants you to be happy (the best men do), and simply state your case: "I don't want to do that, thanks." No, you won't sound rude. You just sound honest and just sound like you don't want to do that, thanks. Simple. Then he'll suggest something else or ask you what you would like to do. Tell him. He should be pleased that you are giving him a chance to make you happy.

A word about appearing rude

"I couldn't refuse because I'd look rude."
"I have to call him, or else I'll seem rude."
"I had to marry him, he'd bought me a ring, so now I live with him and his nine stepchildren because I didn't want to look rude."

Don't worry, you will never seem rude. Think about it, when you like a man and he doesn't phone you, do you think he's being rude? No. You think he's being busy, or caught up with work, or that you're repulsive to all men. "Rude" never comes into it. Or it shouldn't. (If you've called him eight times in a row and he hasn't called back, you're the rude one for pestering the poor man.)

It's strange. This obsession we often have with rudeness is completely out of step with the rest of our lives, where manners have died completely. We never seem to care about being rude when we don't send people thank-you letters, or "forget" to tip waiters, or bring cheap bottles of wine to dinner parties. If you don't want to seem rude, call your mother just to say hello, thank the person on the phone who's taking your message, tip the garbagemen at Christmas. But do not sleep with unappreciative men, agree to lame-ass dates or call your boyfriend every minute of every day. "Rude" actually means offensive or disgusting. It does not mean having your own life or making that life a priority. Okay? I'm glad we got that sorted out.

Dinner at your place

There will come a time early on in a relationship when you want to treat him to dinner at your place. This is a golden opportunity for you to show him how sexy, accomplished and SASSy you are. It's also a very good way to start The Date That Will End With The First Night Together. So don't do this until you've known him a while. Like three months. (I'm serious. Rushing into the bedroom, or the kitchen too soon will only lead to tears later. Don't try too hard too soon.) Here's how to do it with style:

1. Sex up your apartment

If you have roommates, get rid of them for the evening (with plenty of warning). You need to be alone so he can soak up your incredible charms with no diversions. Then clean the entire place from top to bottom. Do this the day before. (I always used to skip this step, thinking I'd just light dim candles and let the darkness be my cleaning lady. I was wrong. The first night my husband-to-be saw my apartment, I'd left fake-tanning streaks on the toilet rim. They were brown, sticky and incredibly hard to explain. I got away with it, but now I clean up for everyone, even the cleaner.)

2. De-angst your bookshelves

Men always head straight for the bookshelves when they come to a woman's home. Perhaps they're just nosy, or perhaps they're looking for books you have in common, but they always do.

So be in no doubt, he will spot any relationship or self-help books you have lurking there, which is obviously bad news for all concerned. Try to get into the habit of keeping all these books in a secret place, and preferably covering them in plain paper. Nothing throws away your mystique faster than your potential partner finding *Women Who Love Prisoners*, *Lose Ten Pounds in Ten Seconds* and *Coping With Self-Hatred* crammed in your bookshelves.

While you're at it, make sure you de-medicine your bathroom, too. Remember you're trying to appear healthy and sexy, so clear the cabinets of any hemorrhoid or yeast-infection creams, antidepressants, cellulite remedies and sanitary products (Extra Absorbent for Torrential Flow). And make sure you remove anything that looks even vaguely stuffed or cuddly or cute from your bedroom (unless it's a sex toy, in which case save it for after dessert).

3. Leave *objets de tart* lying around

Like, a sexy sheer nightie hanging on the back of the bathroom door, so he sees it when he uses your bathroom. He'll imagine you wearing it, which might make it a little difficult to pee for a while. Ahem. Buy yourself a huge bouquet of flowers and have it crammed casually in a vase. Don't tell him who it's from. (He's bound to ask.) Fill your mantelpiece up with party invitations, thank-you cards, photographs — signs of a life being led.

4. Cook a man-friendly meal

Men like meals that look big, include meat (unless he's a vegetarian, of course) and that you don't sweat over. The more trouble he thinks you took over the meal, the less he'll think it was worth it. Guys appreciate that you have a life outside them, and will think you're smart rather than stingy to have used a few ready-to-eat items in your feast.

So ... choose something from the following sample menus, or make up your own versions. Just keep it simple, please. The way to a man's heart isn't through his stomach, it's through your backbone, so don't cook yourself into an early menopause.

Examples of sexy "man meals"

Starter:
King prawns sizzling in garlic butter: You can buy these, with the butter. Have a few torn salad leaves showing wilting on the edge of the plate. Chunky bread for him (not you—wheat bloats the stomach). Garlic isn't a problem if you both eat it.
Or
Ready-to-eat individual Camembert cheeses, breadcrumbed: Bake them for 10 minutes in the oven. Serve with salad and cranberry jelly.

Or
Ready-to-eat smoked salmon pâté served with cream cheese, lemon wedges, capers and mini-toasts. Lay out the pâté and cheese with lemon wedges and capers. Sprinkle with chopped parsley and serve chilled with toast. You can prepare a day ahead.

Main course:
Flash-fried steaks: With more salad, and a baked potato with sour cream and chives.
Or
Spaghetti with lemon and parmesan: Cook spaghetti. When it's drained, add the juice and grated rind of two lemons, a good big handful of grated parmesan, some chopped parsley, salt and pepper. Stir until cheese has melted and pile onto warm plates.
Or
Chicken in red wine served on bed of mashed potatoes: Sauté 1 tbsp garlic in oil in large skillet for two minutes, then add 4 chicken breasts. Cook for about 10 minutes on each side. Sprinkle chicken with 1 tbsp paprika and 1 cup brown sugar, and pour on 1 cup of red wine. Cover, and simmer about 20 minutes. Season to taste with salt and pepper and serve on a bed of mashed potatoes. Tastes gorgeous!

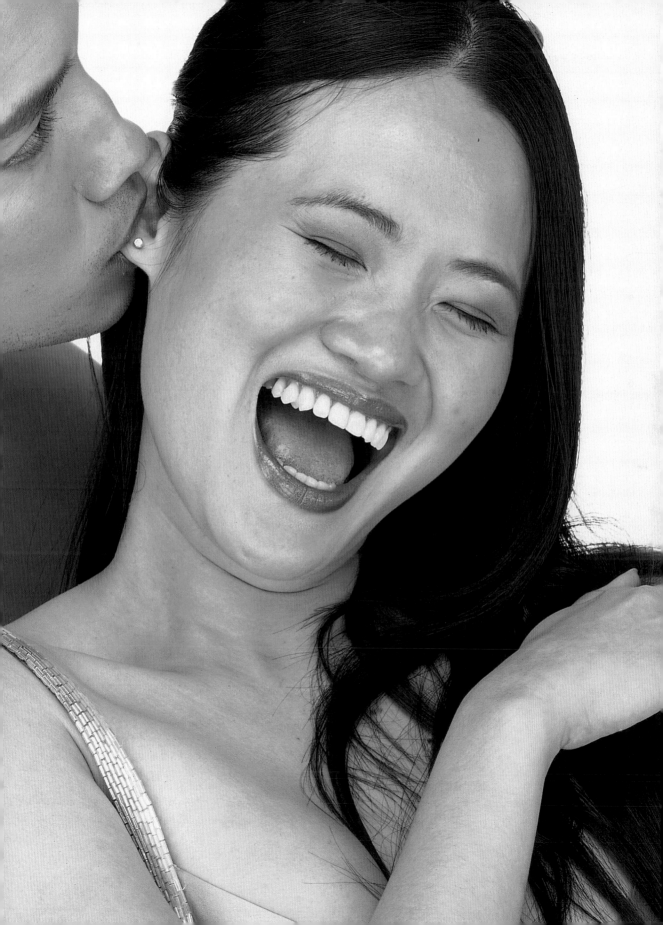

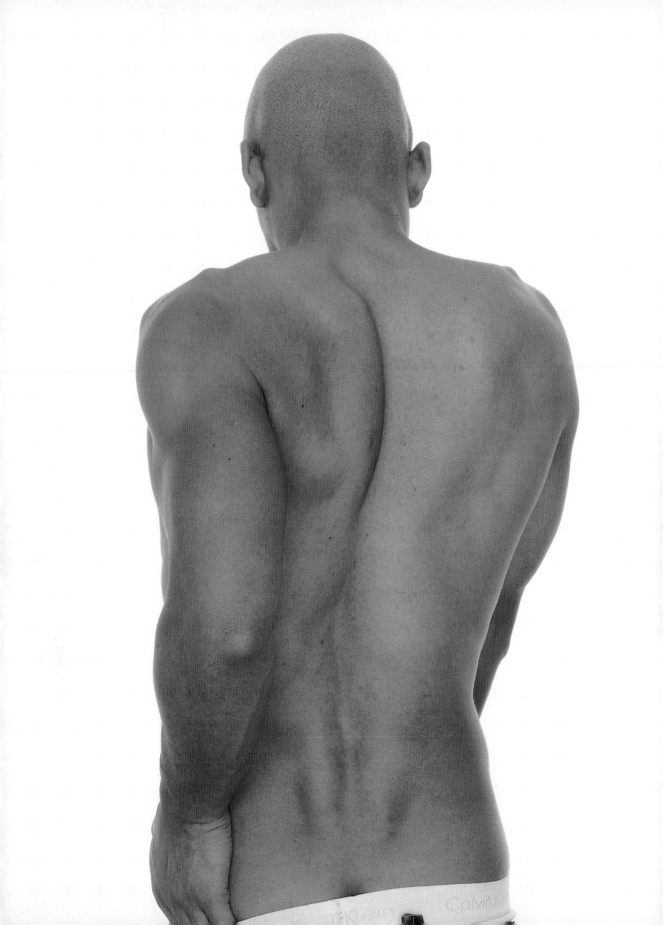

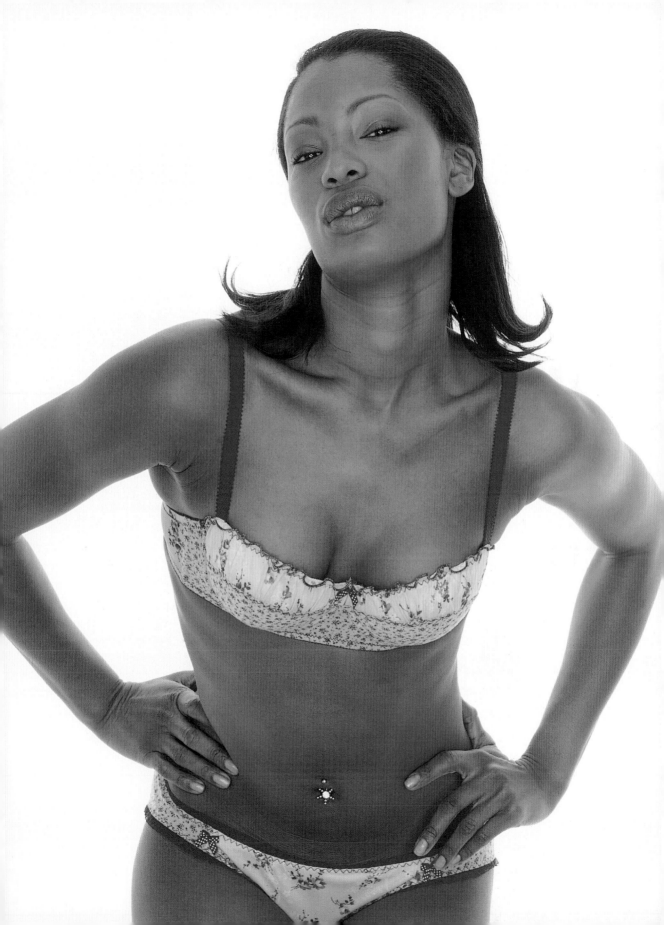

When you decide to cook him
dinner at your place remember to
make light food that will neither
intimidate him nor bloat him. Think
of eating together as foreplay and
your taste buds being the first parts
of your body to get aroused.

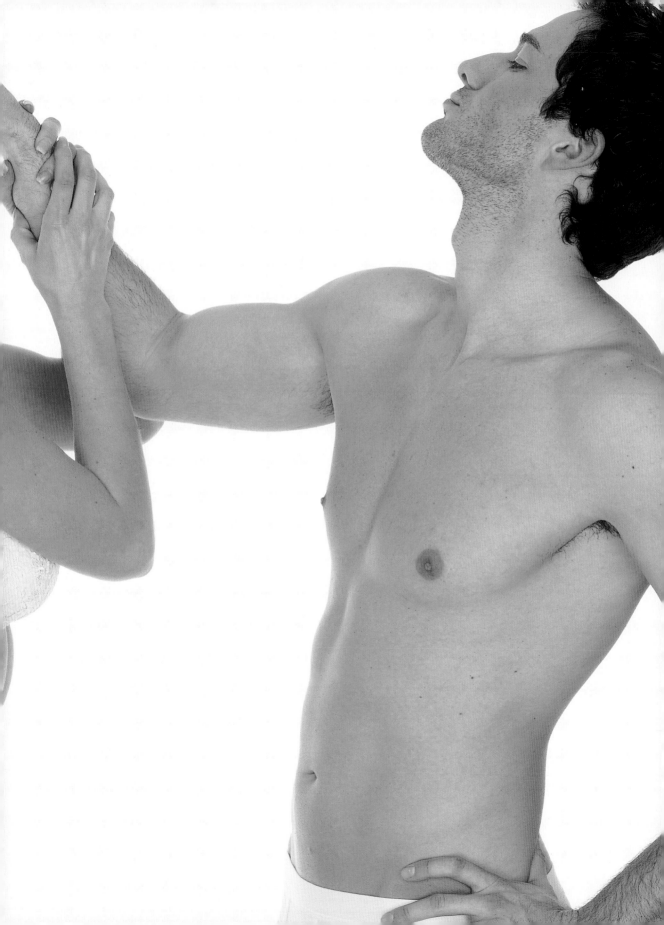

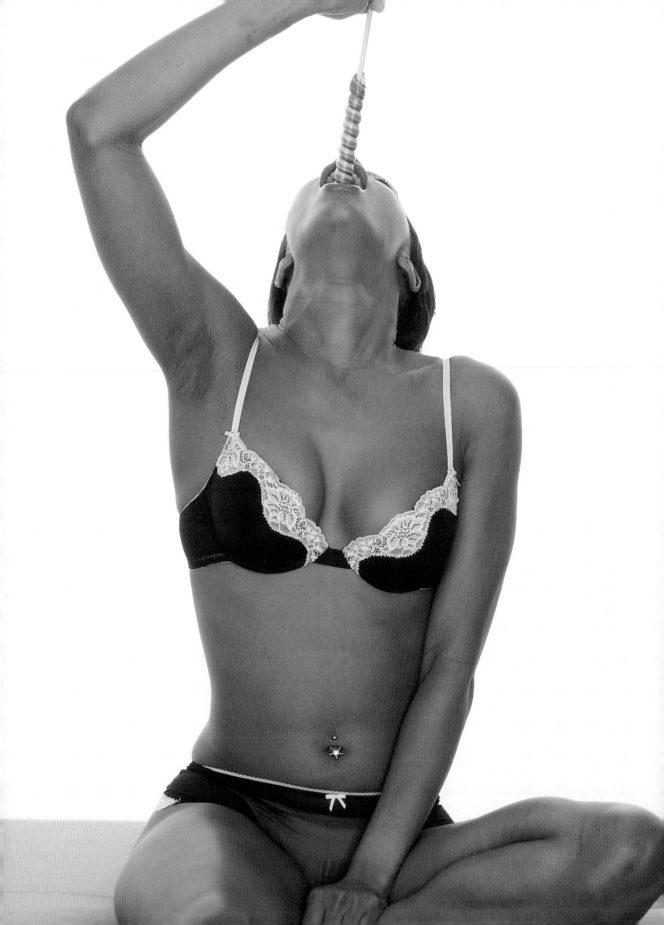

Dessert:

Frozen berries with white-chocolate sauce:
Buy a bag of frozen mixed summer fruits—
raspberries, blueberries, etc. Keep frozen until
time to serve. Pile into dishes. Make sauce by
gently microwaving 1 large bar fine white
chocolate until melted, then stirring in half a
cup of whipping cream. Pour over berries and
serve. Looks very elegant.

Or

Ready-to-eat tiramisu: Add fresh raspberries
to side of dish and dust with icing sugar.

Or

You, served on a bed.

5. As you eat

Remember that sex is never great on a full
stomach, so don't chow down like a starving
refugee. I don't believe in that silly "women
should eat like birds" mantra (as anyone who's
seen me naked will testify), because men are
usually turned on by watching a woman get
sensual pleasure from food—but this is not
the time. So, eat slowly, and with your fingers
where possible. Men love to see your fingers
going towards your mouth!

After the meal, leave it to him to make the
first move. Don't leap on him as soon as he's
had coffee. I know it's old-fashioned but sex
is still best when it's initiated by the man.
This way, he feels in control, and he'll give you
more foreplay—I promise! If he feels like the

sex was his idea, he'll feel it's his job to ensure
you enjoy it. If you leap on him, he'll be much
more passive.

Then just have fun, and leave the dishes in
the sink. You'll have much better uses for those
rubber gloves in the bedroom …

Q+A

■ I can only flirt with men I don't find attractive. Why is this?

■ I just met a man. Should I play hard to get?

● This is because it's easier, as you're not goal-oriented with ugly men. You don't care if they're not attracted to you, so you can be yourself. You need to boost your confidence so you can be ballsy with any man. Get a makeover, have a haircut, buy some new clothes. If you feel that you're looking good, you'll be less shy.

● No. You should *be* hard to get. Fill up your life with friends, work, interests, shopping, clubs, reading, knitting, poker, puppies ... Whatever puts the light behind your eyes. That way he'll get the very best of you—happy, occupied you—and you won't be so likely to worry about the relationship. Some women think they should show their new man just how much of a priority he is from the moment they meet him, but think about it: what do you find sexy? The most attractive man is the distracted, busy man; the scariest is the one who focuses solely on you. Think how previous partners have been unable to keep their hands off you when you're ignoring them. Always put your interests and your life ahead of your boyfriend.

If you don't like the idea of a man deciding *after* sex if he wants you

■ **I share an apartment with a girlfriend. She is obsessed with men and has filled our bookshelves with self-help nonsense. Any man who comes over will think all this stuff is mine. Help!**

● Ask her to move those books into her room. Tell her you've seen friends eyeing up the titles with derision. Tell her it's sexier if her problems are out of sight. If she refuses, hang a sheer voile curtain over the bookcase. It'll look pretty and no man would have the nerve to move it back to check. At least, not on a first date. After that time, you'll know a man well enough to confess that your roommate is a man-crazy loony-tune, and that all the books are hers. This will give the added bonus of making sure he never flirts with her.

■ **Should I ring him the day after we first have sex?**

● I wouldn't. That looks rather clingy. It also signals to him that you are prepared to do a lot of the work in the relationship, and that you're committed to making a proper go of it. That isn't actually a very good idea. After sex, men relax and, sadly, often spend time deciding whether they actually want to be in a committed sexual relationship with you. Don't interrupt that time with calls. Give him time to think about what happened and, when he's ready, he'll ring you. If you don't like the idea of a man deciding after sex if he wants you, hold out for as long as possible before you go to bed with him. Then he'll have made the decision *before* you hit the mattress.

hold out for as long as possible *before* you go to bed with him.

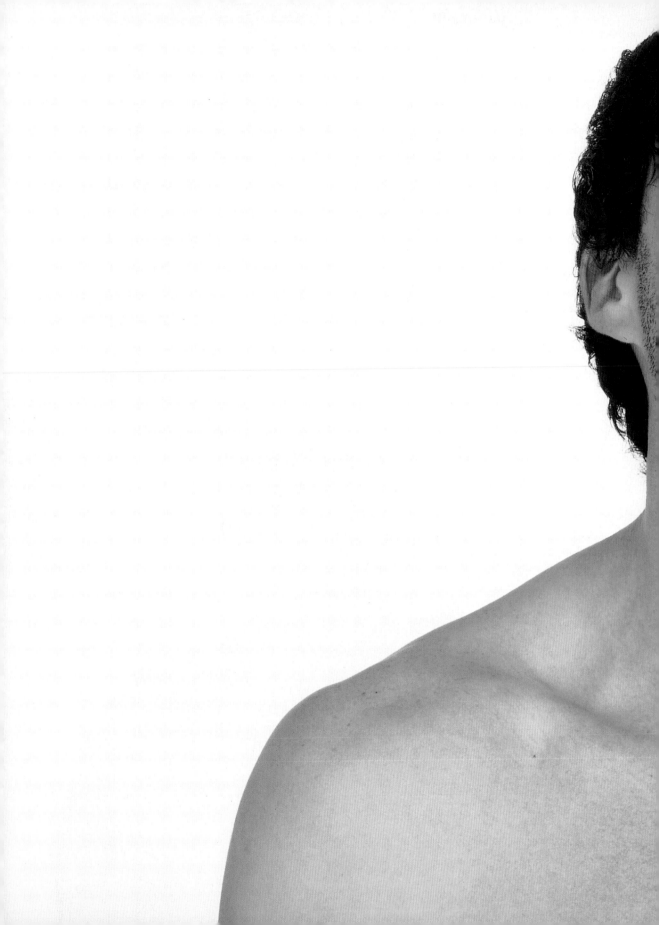

3 Handy hints

(have him eating out of the palm of your hand)

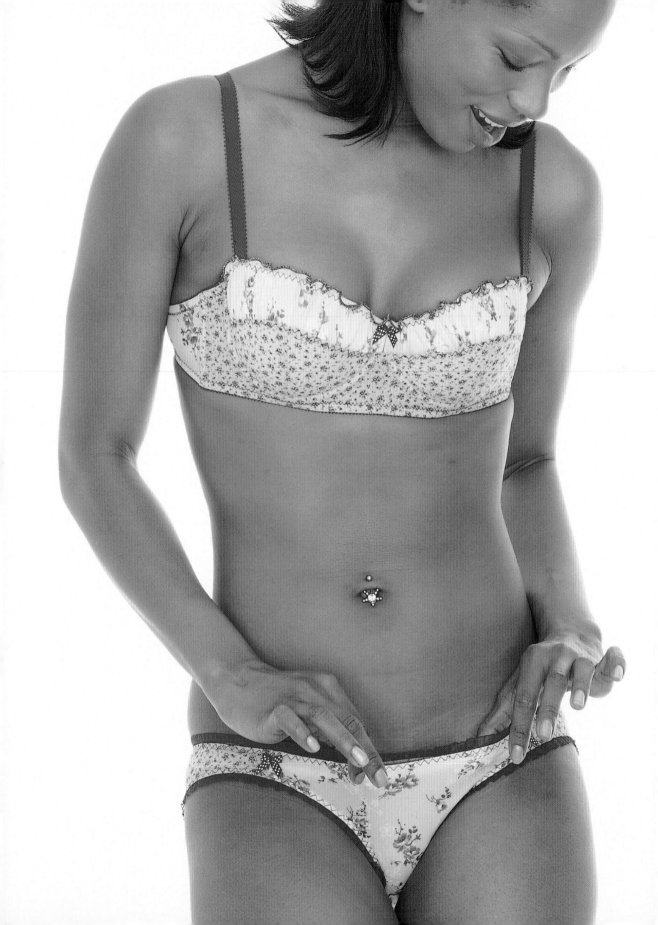

Personal story: Imagine it's your penis

I **was never very good with my hands.** It's just so hard to imagine what a penis would respond to, not having one myself. Eventually, a boyfriend gave me a copy of a sex book. He gave it to me as a present, but it was a present for him really. I was a bit offended but I read it avidly.

The best tip in the book was to imagine that the dick was mine. The author said to hold the penis in one hand and close my eyes and try to feel what the penis was feeling. He said it would be a good way to "understand" the dick; to know what type of stroke would be most exciting. The first time I tried that, the boyfriend was ecstatic. It made me change my stroke—I'd been gripping the dick quite tightly before; now, I loosened my grip and tried to caress it, instead of choking it like a dead chicken.

Blow jobs were harder to master. There's so much to do at once: like rubbing your stomach and patting your head simultaneously. The book said that men love it when women swallow. I can understand that, it's much sexier than having a woman run to the bathroom, coughing and sputtering. I'd hate it if a man refused to go down on me because of my feminine fluids. But even so, I could never bear to swallow this boyfriend's semen. When he got close to coming, he'd grip my head in his hands and really push it down onto his penis. It's a shock, sometimes, when it erupts into your mouth. And it can taste funny, depending on what he's eaten. They didn't mention that in the book.

I finished with the boyfriend eventually, but I kept the book. I used to refer to it from time to time to brush up on my skills. Nowadays I've got my oral technique down to quite a fine art. I start off by teasing the dick for a while—sort of stroking all around it, leaving the actual shaft till last. I've noticed that when men do the same to me—not touching my vagina for ages—it concentrates the sensation in that area. All I can feel is my vagina, just aching to be touched. So I do the same to men.

I've had several men tell me that I give really good head and it's all down to that little book.

Sarah, 41

Hello girls

So, here we go. This is, in some ways, the most important chapter in the book because if you can give a man a brilliant blow job, he'll be yours forever. I know that you're dying to learn BJ tricks, because it's the one question I get asked over and over again by women. I've even had someone famous ask me for tips—I'd love to tell you who, but I can't. Just know that it was someone who you'd have thought would already know everything …

Before we begin, I'm going to give you a guided tour of the penis. It's essential, because you have to know all of his hotspots if you intend to get him really hot. Arousing your man before you perform specific sexual techniques is crucial—it's the sexual equivalent of getting your dinner-party guests drunk before you serve the meal. If he's incredibly horny (or, actually, incredibly drunk) he won't notice if you mess up a bit.

Know his private parts

1. The glans

This is what you see when you roll back the foreskin. The tip of the penis is very, very sensitive, containing billions and billions of nerve endings.
Likes: Licking and gentle sucking.
Dislikes: Fingernails, overly enthusiastic tongue-flicking, being stimulated immediately after ejaculation.

2. The coronal ridge

The bit at the bottom of the glans that sticks out. Very sensitive.
Likes: Having a tongue run around it; being licked underneath.
Dislikes: Teeth. Ouch.

3. The shaft

The main body of the penis. It contains three spongy erectile caverns that fill with blood, causing an erection. As far as your pleasure is concerned, how *long* this part is doesn't matter as much as how *wide* it is. Remember, the underneath of his shaft (the side nearest his legs) is the most sensitive part. Direct most of your pressure there.
Likes: Being gripped with medium pressure—hold it as hard as you'd hold a can of Coke. Not so hard that you'd crush it (ouch), but not so light that you'd drop it.
Dislikes: Being squeezed hard, or being touched with irritating, too-light butterfly touches. If you're going to hold it, *hold* it.

4. The frenulum

A good Scrabble word and a highly sensitive part of the penis. This is the piece of skin that connects the foreskin (if he has one) to the shaft of the penis. Its colloquial name is a "banjo string."
Likes: Being held between your lips, being sucked, sucking and humming.

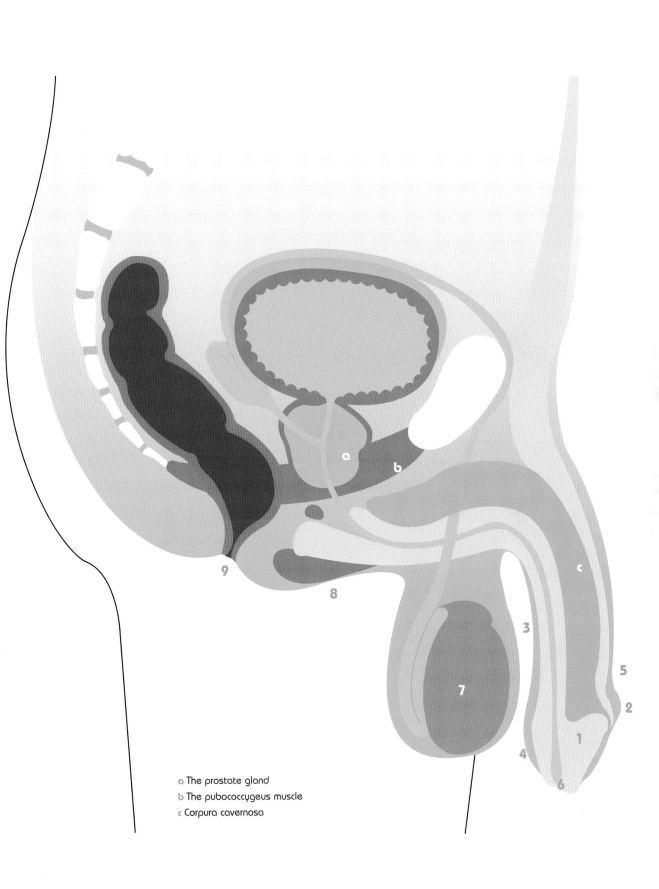

a The prostate gland
b The pubococcygeus muscle
c Corpura cavernosa

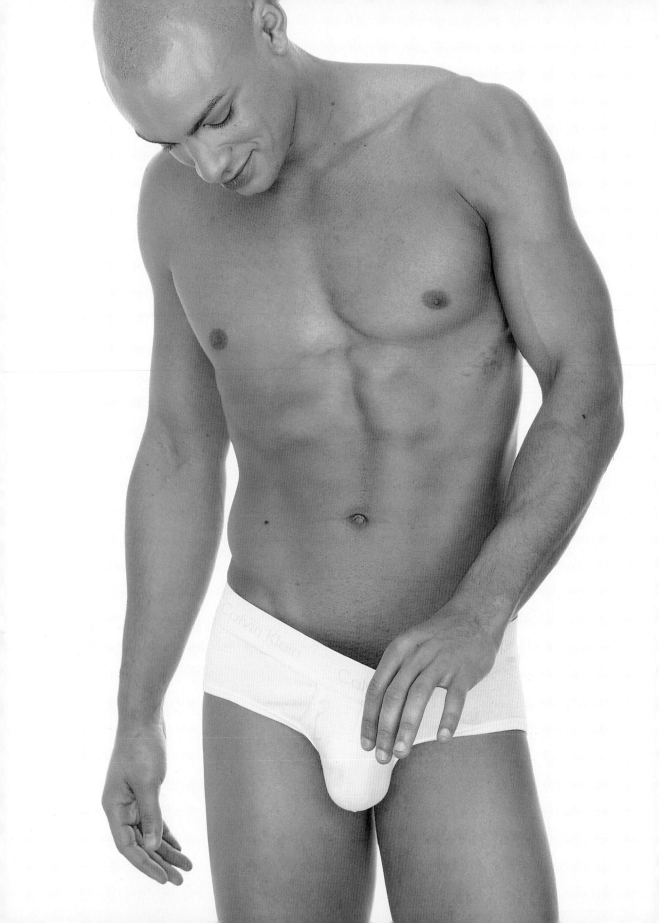

Dislikes: Being plucked as if it were a banjo string. Note: the frenulum can split during rough sex, but it's not an emergency. Honest.

5. The foreskin

Not sensitive on its own, this bit of skin covering the top of the penis is useful for stimulating the head of the penis. In sex, this rubs up and down over the glans with the friction of his thrusts, and feels good.
Likes: Being slid back with your tongue.
Dislikes: Being pulled or stretched. Not a real hotspot, so don't give it too much attention, aside from pushing it back.

6. The urethral opening

This is the opening of the penis that lets out urine and semen, and pre-come. Sensitive.
Likes: Being licked, or having the tip of your tongue swirled around it. Some men like having the tip of a tongue gently (so gently) inserted into the opening. Ask first.
Dislikes: Having anything pushed down it.

7. The scrotum

The sack that contains the testes. Usually loose, but retracts when the man is aroused, startled or cold. Handle with care: very sensitive.
Likes: Being cupped, stroked, fondled, licked. Some men can't get enough of having their balls sucked. The skin is even more sensitive than the testicles inside, so concentrate your efforts accordingly.
Dislikes: Being squeezed, tugged or accidentally bashed. Agony.

8. The perineum

The area between the testicles and the anus. Loaded with nerve endings, and almost as sensitive as the penis itself. The prostate gland can also be stimulated by applying pressure to the perineum.
Likes: Massage, stroking, licking.
Dislikes: Being jabbed or poked.

9. The anus

In case you don't know, this is the opening of the rectum. Very sensitive to the touch, as it's surrounded by both nerves and fine hairs, which make it very receptive to your advances. Swells during arousal. Inside the anus is the prostate gland, which is often called the male G-spot. Incredibly sensitive to the touch, in fact can cause spontaneous ejaculation.
Likes: Being licked, probed.
Dislikes: Fingernails, cheap toilet paper.

Now what?

Okay. So you've got to know his penis. But what should you do with it? Here we go.

You have to know all his hotspots and what to do with them

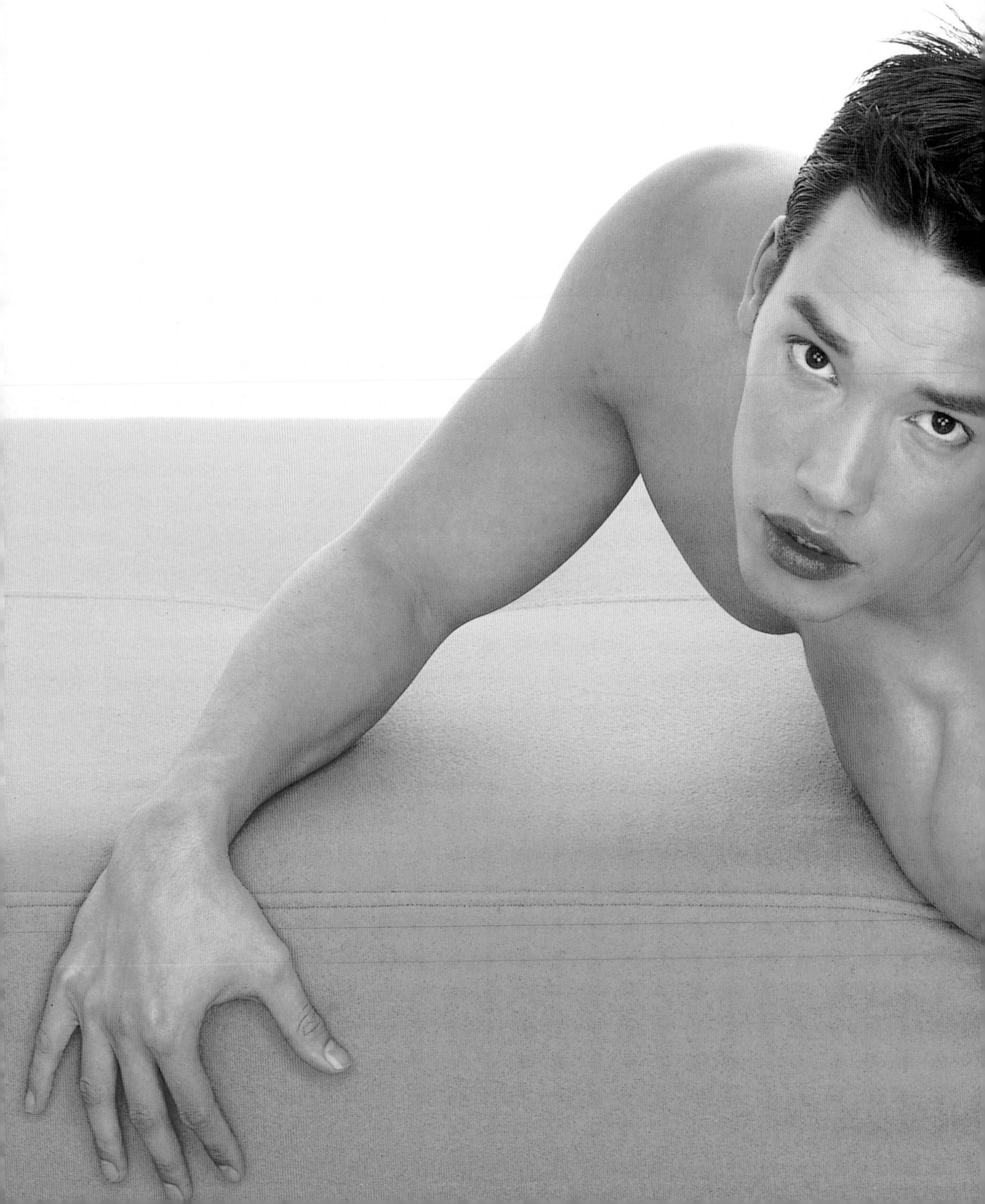

if you really want to make him go wild.

How to give the perfect blow job

Step 1: Arouse him

You want to get him as horny as possible before you go anywhere near his private parts. The reason is simple: the more aroused he is, the better everything's going to feel. You know when you're really turned on, that first touch on your privates nearly blows your head off? That's the sensation you want to recreate.

The easiest and best arousal technique is kissing. Nothing hardens a male faster than a good, hard kiss. Kiss his face off, and start stroking him all around—but not on—his penis. Start kissing downward, over his body. (Tip: Does he spend a lot of time sucking your nipples? If so, it may be that he has sensitive nipples himself. People often do to their partner what they'd like to have done to them. If so, lick his nipples and suck on the buds.) When you get near to his penis, it should soon be obvious how turned on he is. Don't be insulted if he's still flaccid; it takes some men longer to get hard than others.

Step 2: Assume the position

Push him on the bed, lying on his back. Kneel in between his knees and lick your way over one inner thigh, along his perineum, and back up the other inner thigh. He'll love this, as your hair will be tickling his penis and balls. Repeat a couple of times. Swirl your tongue along the skin over his hipbones—very hot—and then down … down …

Step 3: Grasp the shaft

Now you should have his penis in your face. Frightening, aren't they, up close? Grasp the shaft in one hand. Curl your fingers around it, and hold it with medium pressure. (If the head bulges—or his eyes do, you are too firm.) See the vein running down underneath? Press your thumb on it, gently. That side of the penis is the most sensitive, so run your thumb along it.

Step 4: Pull back the foreskin

Stroke down with that hand until the foreskin (if he has one) is pulled back. Now the head of his penis is exposed and, if he's very excited, it might be already leaking some pre-come.

Step 5: Lick the tip

Bend your head over it, and lightly lick all over the top. He should groan. Keep licking the very tip, like you're licking a delicately balanced ice-cream cone. Then lick down, all around the coronal ridge. This is so, so hot for him. He should start to thrash—and I bet seeing him in that state is doing it for you too by now.

Step 6: Mind those molars

We're going in now, so cover your teeth with your lips. Still holding the shaft, lower your head and slide his penis into your mouth. Run your tongue all over it, up and down the sides, really swirl it around. Get the saliva going. Move your head up and down, sucking gently.

Killer move no. 1: Wet your hand

When you have a mouth full of saliva, take his penis out of your mouth and wet the palm of your hand with it. Then hold his penis again. He'll love the feeling of your wet hand stroking his cock. Go back to sucking on him, running your hand up and down his shaft. Make sure you keep rewetting the hand when it dries out.

Killer move no. 2: Finger and thumb ring

With the other hand, form your finger and thumb into a ring. Place it around his penis, just underneath the coronal ridge. Place your lips just above it. Now move both hands up and down, keeping your finger-ring underneath your lips all the time. The ring will feel like an extension of your mouth.

Step 7: Quicken the pace

Now start to increase the pace, always keeping both hands moving up and down, and bobbing your head up and down at the same time. Suck his dick. Then try to create a kind of "vagina" with your mouth, by making sure that the insides of your cheeks rub his shaft. (Tip: Don't worry about him going in too deep. Yes, men like it when you can get as much of their penis in your mouth as possible, but using your hands, and your finger-ring will trick him into thinking he's much farther into your mouth than he really is.)

Step 8: Making him come

By this time you may be worried about lockjaw, so you want to make him come. Keep both hands moving and keep sucking. Speed up a bit more. You could tickle his balls with one hand; that usually induces orgasm. Or lean forward and let your breasts tickle his balls and penis. He'll appreciate visuals, so ensure your hair isn't covering your face. Let him see what you're doing. Look at him while you do it.

Signs he's about to come

He may tell you. His balls will tighten and rise up closer to his body. He may produce more pre-come. His breathing will increase and he'll get noisier. He'll thrust his hips upwards.

Coming!

He'll go, "Oh, oh, oh, oh ... " Or his actions will build up to some climax. Or he'll tell you. Depending on what you prefer, your options are:
- He can come in your mouth. If you don't like the taste, try to get his penis right to the back of your throat. That way the semen will run down your throat and you won't taste it.
- He can come over your face. Pull his penis out at the very last second and let him spurt onto your face. Close your eyes.
- He can watch himself come into your mouth. A good compromise: pull his penis out of your mouth, but keep it close enough so the semen pumps onto your tongue.

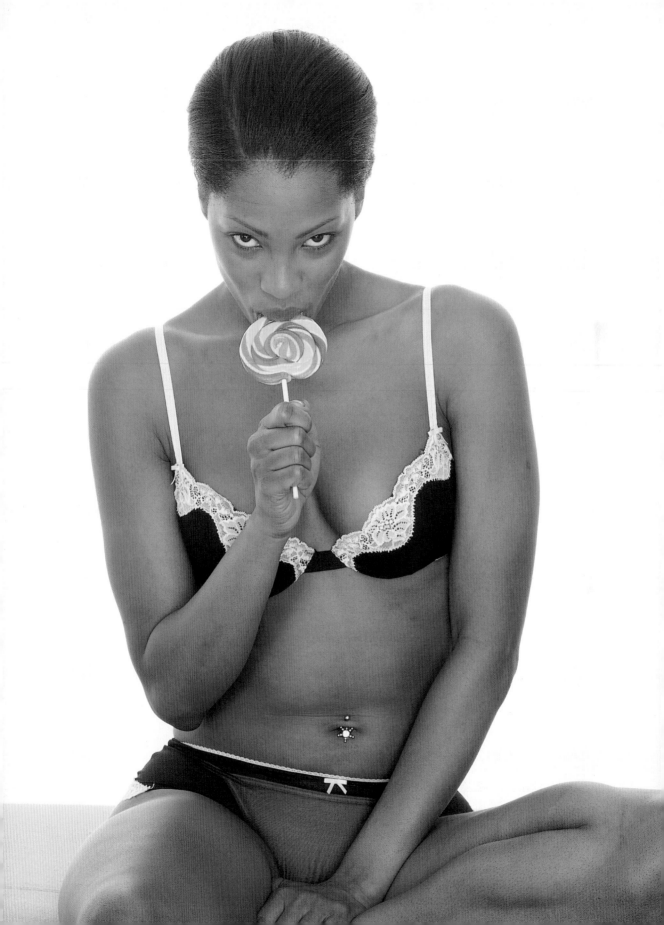

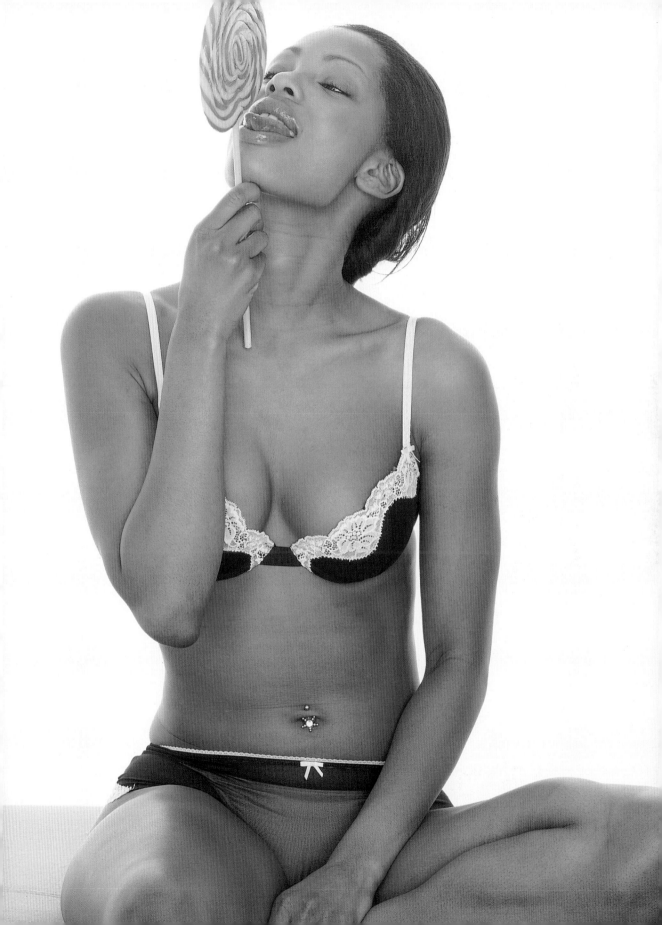

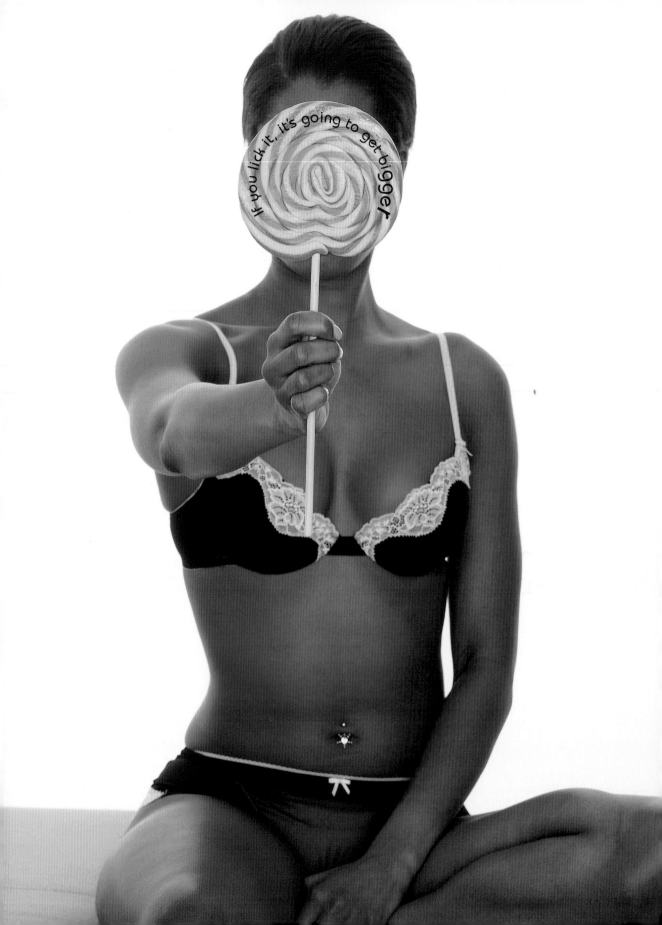

● He can think he's come in your mouth, but he hasn't really. Keep your mouth very slightly open as he comes, and let the semen spill immediately back out again.

● He can come over your chest. Don't forget this option—it's an easy way to avoid a mouthful of semen (if you don't like it) and he'll think it's very sexy to watch. Rub it in like it's body lotion for maximum effect.

Variations

Once you've mastered the basic blow job, you can add variations. Here are some of the best:

Things that make you go hum
When his penis is inside your mouth, hum. Yes you'll feel stupid but it'll feel fabulous—the vibrations will go right through him. Just try it and see. (Tip: if he likes it, have him repay the favor on your clitoris and nipples.)

Corny
Hold his penis sideways in your mouth, as if it were a corn on the cob. "Nibble" up and down with tiny, teeny little bites. Don't actually bite the poor man, just pretend-nibble. Shiversome.

Shake it, baby
Hold his penis in your mouth and shake your head from side to side, like you're saying "No." He'll be saying, "Yes, yes, yes … "

Sweet like chocolate
Cover his penis in something sexy and sweet, like chocolate sauce or flavored body paint, then slowly lick it off. Fattening, but worth it.

Minty fresh
Gargle with a strong mint mouthwash before you hit the sheets. As you suck his penis, he'll feel that minty-coolness all over your mouth. Surprising as it sounds, this is very sexy.

The hot and cold running blow job
Take a break from the basic blow job and drink a mouthful of warm coffee. Swallow, then insert his dick back into your mouth. You'll feel super-warm and he'll love it. If you're feeling more ambitious, you can alternate with sips of iced water. Hot/cold, hot/cold—hot!

Phone sex
Next time he is on the phone to his boss or the bank manager, sneak up to his private parts and start giving him the sexiest blow job you can give. It'll feel extra naughty and "not allowed"—which he'll love.

Wake me up before you come, come
A very common male fantasy is being woken up in the middle of the night with a blow job. What are you waiting for? Hopefully you'll then be woken up with that common female fantasy—breakfast in bed.

Stand and deliver

I've known many men whose number-one favorite sex act was the standing blow job. He stands in front of you, and you kneel down and "worship" his dick. He likes it because he gets a great view of his dick sliding in and out of your mouth; you like it because it's comfy, and you can play with every inch of him. (Tip: cup his balls while you do it. They're extra-sensitive when they're hanging down.)

Dong in cheek

Push his penis into the side of your cheek as you suck him. It'll feel, to him, like he's going in really deep. This is also a good way to give yourself a break from hard sucking if your jaw is aching.

How to deep throat

Have you ever seen this famous porn film? It's the story of a woman whose clitoris is in the back of her throat. Ergo, she can only orgasm when she is sucking a man's dick. All together now, "Aaaah." *Bambi* it ain't. But we can use it to our advantage if we learn from it. What can we learn? That ramming a cock deep into a woman's neck is about the sexiest thing in the world for a man, ever.

If you've never deep-throated (and very few women have) you'll be terrified. You fear you won't be able to breathe, or you'll choke, or you'll vomit all over your bedside table. Truth?

You won't, if you follow the guidelines below. It's a way of deep-throating that is extremely easy to do.

Lie down on your back on the bed. Hang your head over the edge, so that your mouth and throat form a straight line. This will "open" the back of your throat, so you can take his penis in very deeply.

He should stand beside the bed and slowly feed his penis into your mouth. Take a deep breath: as his penis goes deeper, it's going to block your breathing. Don't panic! When he pulls it out again, you can take another deep breath. It's actually quite easy once you've got the hang of it.

Safe signal

Before you begin, let him know that deep-throating can be dangerous if he goes too deep for too long. Agree on a "safe signal" beforehand: this is an action that you can perform that tells him to stop immediately. A good signal is to bang your hand on the bed three times. If he sees you do that, he must withdraw his penis immediately. Obviously, don't try anything that you don't feel comfortable with, especially with a new partner.

How to 69

A friend of mine once sent a Valentine to a man she liked, with the touching message: "Wine me, dine me, 69 me." Did he respond? Like a

How to give the perfect hand job

shot. It's another male fantasy. Here's how to do it so he'll remember you forever—and never forget Valentine's Day:

● He lies on the bed, on his back. Place a small pillow or cushion underneath his neck: you want to give him lots of support so he can raise his head off the bed and get himself right into you.

● Straddle his body, facing his feet, until your vagina is hovering over his mouth. Start by teasing him—trail your fingernails over his thighs, kiss his hips, run a tongue close to (but not over) his dick. When he pulls your bottom down to start licking your vagina, slide his penis into your mouth. It'll be the opposite way around to how you usually approach it, so remember that its most sensitive side (the underneath) is now on the top. Lick and suck as described in "How to Give the Perfect Blow Job."

Then tell him to slide his tongue deeply into your vagina. When he does, grip it and hold it there with your PC muscles. Now make your mouth and vagina contract simultaneously—your mouth pulses around his penis as your vagina pulses around his tongue. Keep going for as long as you both can take the heat!

Tip: A good variation on the 69 is to alternate your mouth with your vagina. In between sucks, shift forwards and sink his penis into your vagina. Do it like that for a few seconds, then return to the starting position. Keep mixing up the moves like that and he won't know if he's coming, or coming.

This is a very underrated skill. Underrated by women, that is. Men adore hand jobs. Probably not as much as a blow job, but it comes in a close second. The secret is: lubrication. Imagine you had a penis. Would you like it if someone rubbed it fast and hard, with a dry hand? Hmmm? Nope. You'd feel like they were going to start a fire in your pubes. Nasty.

Start like a blow job, but lube up your hand first. You could use saliva but it dries really quickly. The best lubricants come in a pump-top bottle that you can operate with one hand.

So you're all lubed up. Now what? Try these handy hints.

Firestarter

One good way to start a hand job is with this little maneuver. It's a very good way to give him an erection.

Hold his penis between both palms, and roll it. Imagine you're a boy scout trying to light a fire. Go gently, and build up the pressure. Once he's hard that won't feel as good, so move on to something else. Like …

Twist and (he'll) shout

Get him to sit on a chair, or the bed, and you sit down facing him, in between his legs. Don't perch anywhere rickety—this is a slow, sexy hand job that you'll want to keep up for a while. Turn your hand upside down and grip his penis (you should be seeing the back of your hand,

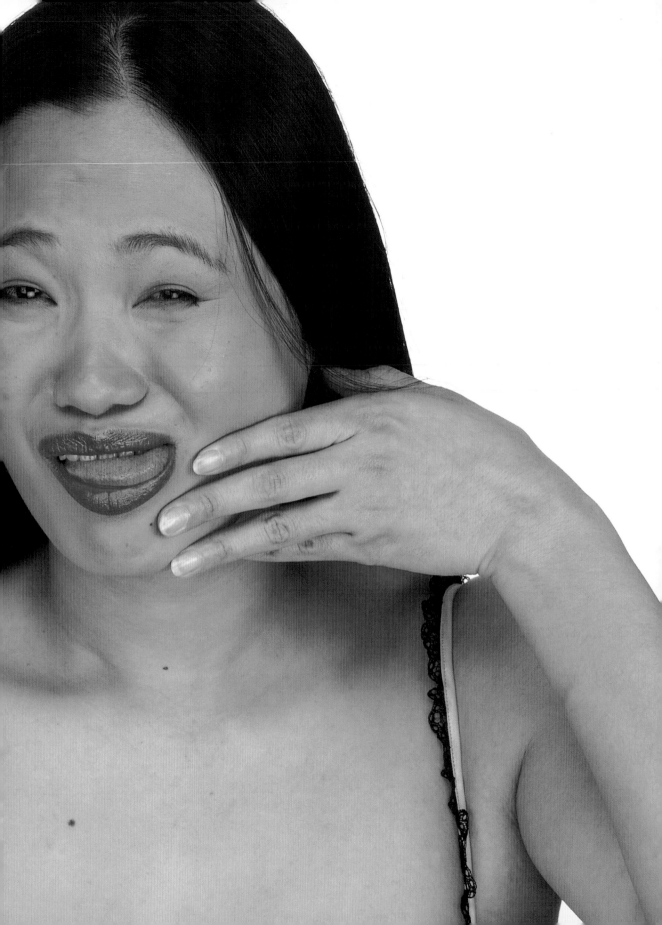

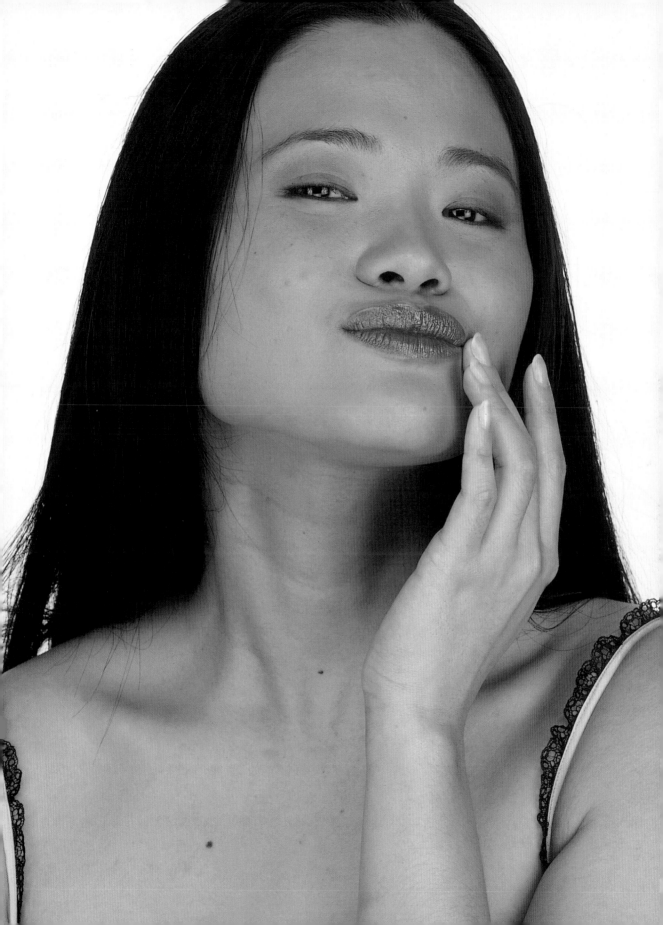

69 is a male fantasy and if you know how to

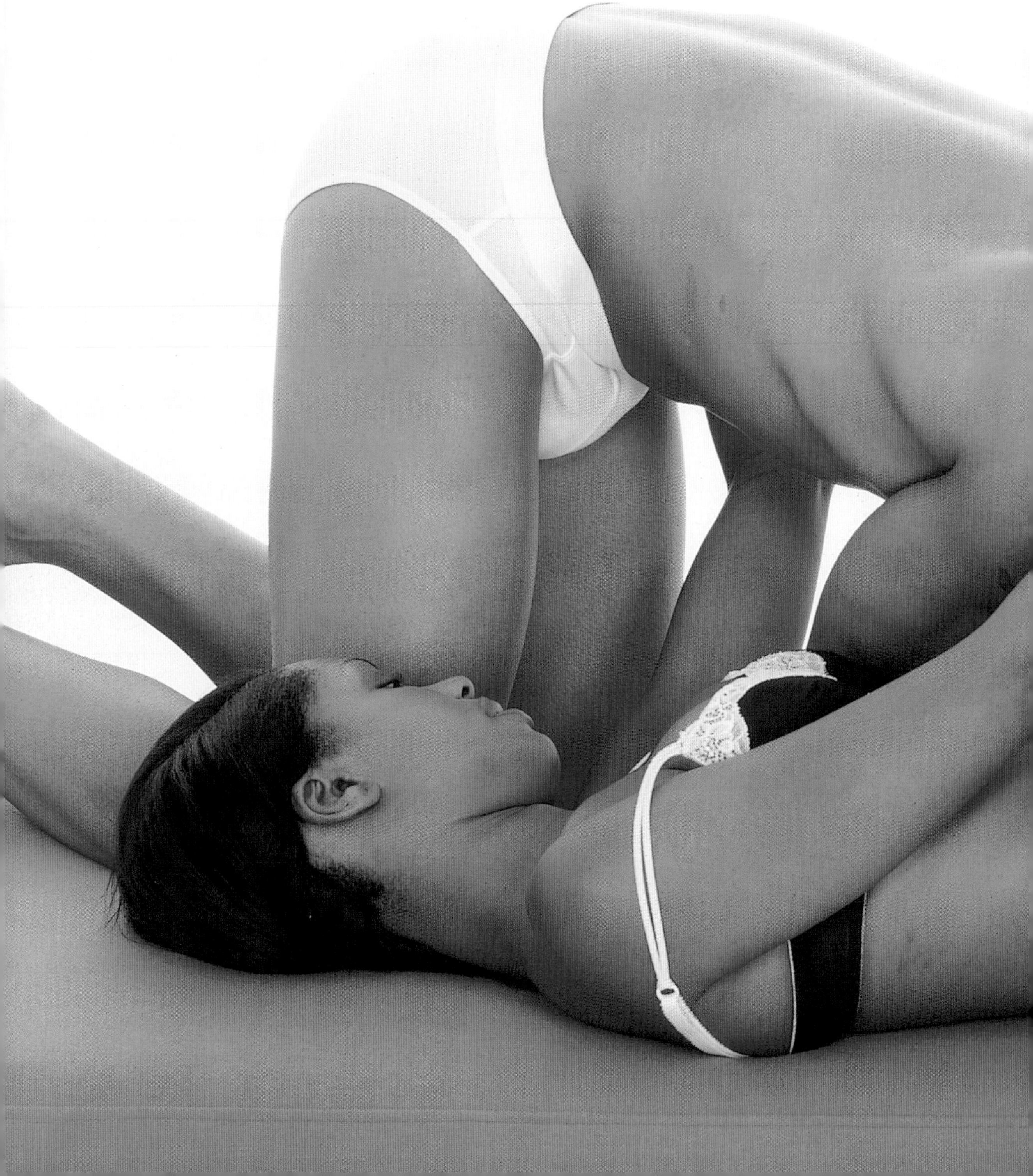

do it properly he will remember you forever.

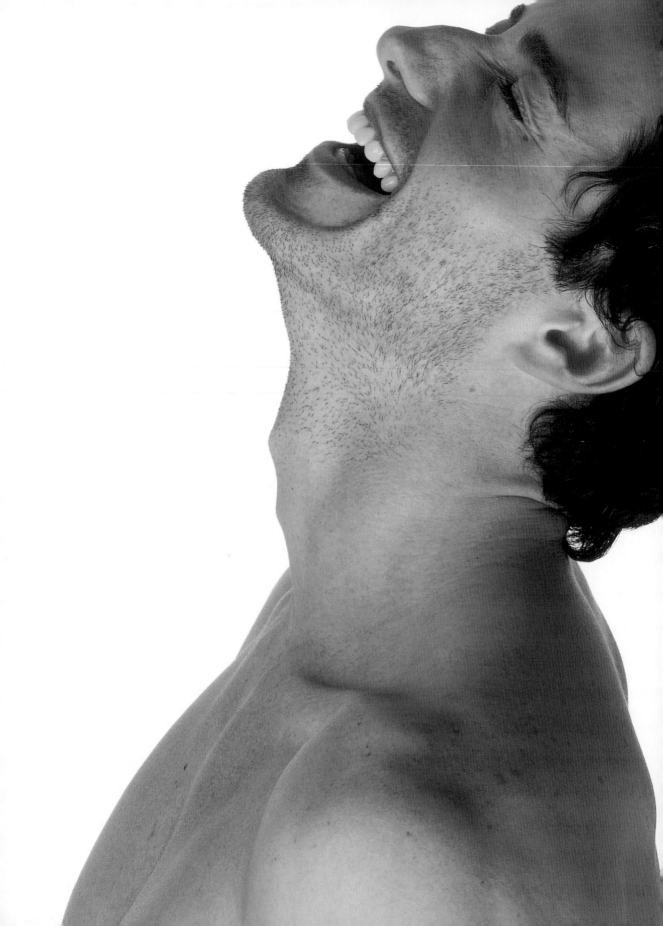

with your thumb at the bottom). With your fingers circling his shaft, move the hand up, slowly twisting around until you reach the top. Then release your fingers and let your palm glide over the head of his penis. Don't lose contact: it's the constant contact of your hand on his meat that makes this feel so good.

Then grip the shaft again—your hand will be facing the other way now, with the fingers nearest you—and slide it back down, twisting again as you go. Repeat the action for as long as he can stand it. Which might not be for long—I learned this trick from a gay man who uses it as his "signature" move. He has men falling over themselves for a date with him. Try it, and you'll have the same.

Basketweave

Lou Paget, the author of *365 Days of Sensational Sex*, is to sex what Ferrari is to cars. She introduced me to this move when she appeared on *Sex Tips for Girls*. The men on the show were all blown away by it. What they loved is that it provides constant friction over every inch of the penis—from the shaft to the head. Try it now.

Start by applying plenty of lubricant to the palms of both hands. Then interlock your fingers and thumbs loosely, so they form a "basket." Slip this over his penis, so the glans pokes out between your thumbs.

Then clasp your hands a little tighter around him; the idea is to form an artificial vagina with your hands. Move them up his penis slowly until you reach the top. When you do, twist your hands back towards you, so your interlocked fingers glide over the head of his penis. Then twist them back down over the head again, and then back down the shaft.

Two hands are better than one

Grip his penis with both hands. Then twist the hands in opposite directions, i.e., one clockwise, one counterclockwise. Then twist them both back again. Keep repeating, perhaps moving your hands up and down his dick as you go. Lovely. If his dick isn't big enough for two hands to hold it, stroke him with one, and use the other to roam around his private parts, tickling his balls, pressing against his perineum, or grasping the base of his penis if he's just about to come.

No mercy no. 1

So called because you never stop the pace— you just keep the strokes coming and coming. Bring one hand down, letting it stroke the penis from the top all the way to the bottom. When it hits the bottom, release it. Meanwhile, bring your other hand to the top of the shaft and stroke down. The strokes just keep following each other, each one bringing him closer to the inevitable thrashing, blissful, intense climax.

No mercy no. 2

As above, but rather than just stroking your hand down his penis, form a fist and let his dick "penetrate" it with each stroke. Before the top of his penis appears out of your fist, have the other hand ready to be penetrated. It feels like he's sinking deeper and deeper into a bottomless vagina … Awesome.

The weenie wiggle

Another terrific trick from a gay man, this move seems scary at first but I can assure you — it doesn't hurt him. What you do is grip his dick with both hands. Imagine you're playing a flute. Grip the loose skin on either side of it. Now, wiggle the penis back and forth, holding on to that skin. As you build up speed, he'll love it.

Squeeze me, please me

Imagine you're going to do the Firestarter (p. 79). Place a hand on each side of his dick. But instead of rolling it between them, press on the shaft from both sides, then move your hands up, then down. It'll pull on the base of his dick, and tug at his balls. And feel amazing.

Hold it!

Form a circle with the finger and thumb of one hand. Grip the base of his penis tightly. This will act like a cock ring, which slows the flow of blood away from his dick and keeps it extra-hard for longer. Now use the other hand

(and loads of lube) to do innumerable rude things to him. Everything will feel super-sexy when he's being held so hard.

Hair we go

Don't forget to play with the pubic hairs that grow on his balls. Lightly pull on them, blow on them, tease them with your fingertips. Very hot.

Thigh's the limit

While you stroke his dick with one hand, use the other to stroke and caress his inner thighs. Look for the place where the hairs are sparse, just below his penis. Very sensitive. Kiss, lick, blow, rub.

Knuckle duster

Form your hand into a fist, and press the knuckles against his perineum. Once he feels what you're up to, he'll open wider to give you better access. The pressure will blow his mind.

Palm springs no. 1

Use your open palm to swirl around the head of his penis. It'll make it harder and even more sensitive to everything you do. Alternate the direction of the swirls for added appeal.

Palm springs no. 2

Like the above, use your open palm on his glans, but stop at each "hour of the clock," and make circular motions with your open palm.

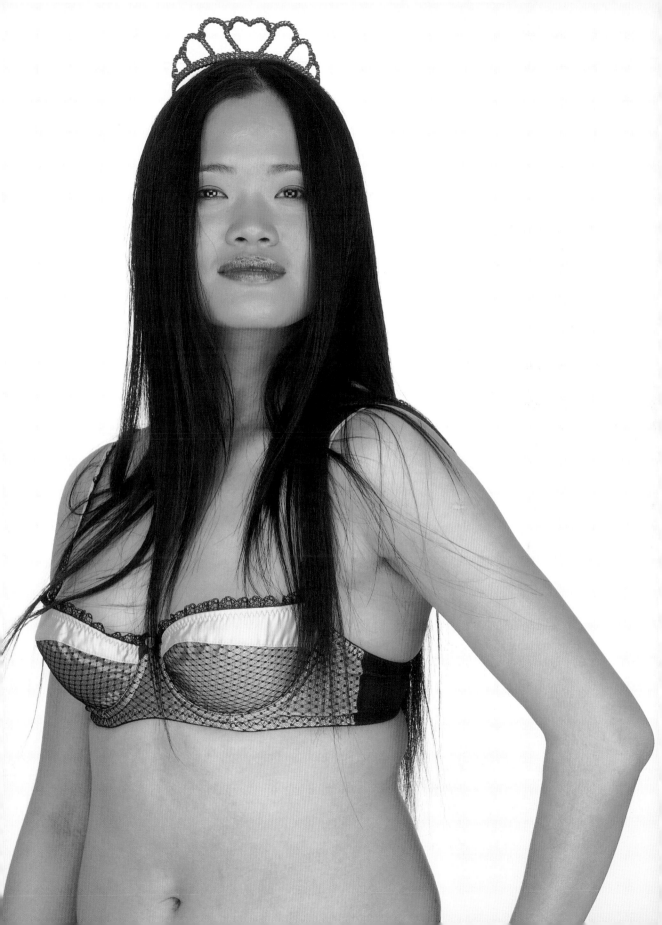

Q+A

■ **When I tried to give my man a hand job, he took over and finished it off himself. I'm so insulted! Should I be?**

■ **My partner has asked for a "boob screw." Help!**

● The thoughtless heathen. He probably just isn't very good at communicating what it is he'd like you to do to him. As he's not embarrassed about jerking off in front of you (as lots of men are), use that to your advantage. Ask him to play with himself while you watch. That way, you can take mental notes on what he does and what he likes, and he'll find it very sexy to be watched. Alternatively, ask him to play with himself while you retire to the living room, kick off your shoes and see what's on TV.

● Loads of men love these but they're a bit fussy, so save it for a special occasion. Birthdays and Christmas, I always say. Okay. Here's what you do: have him kneel on the bed, stroking his (well-lubed) dick. You kneel in front of him and squeeze your breasts together with both hands. He can feed his dick in between your breasts, and thrust in and out. Or you can hold your boobs together with one hand, and use the other to guide his penis in and out. (The second option only works if you have small boobs.) He'll like it because of the friction of your boobs, plus it looks very sexy.

Ask him to play with himself while you watch. That way, you can

■ **Whenever I give my boyfriend a hand job, he comes almost instantly. I don't mind, but we've been together for some time and he says he'd like to enjoy it for longer. What shall I do?**

● See? I told you hand jobs were powerful things. You can help him overcome his excitement in a number of ways:

a. Place your hand flat on the top of his penis and press down very gently.

b. Have him hold the base of his penis tight with one hand when he feels he's about to shoot—this is a good, tried and tested way of delaying orgasm.

c. Stop being so darned sexy, woman.

■ **My jaw aches after mere seconds of giving him a blow job. Any tips?**

● Keep the faith. It will get better the more BJs you perform. But in the meantime, shift your position so that he is lying on his back, with you lying next to him. Lean your head on his hip and give him the blow job that way. It'll ease your jaw, and increase your saliva—it will pool in your mouth. With all that lubrication you can wet your hand and use it to bring him off while your jaw takes a break. Use the tip of a wetted finger for anal teasing. And be thankful you're not a man with a jaw that has to keep going for even longer when he's down on his woman.

ake mental notes on what he does and what he likes.

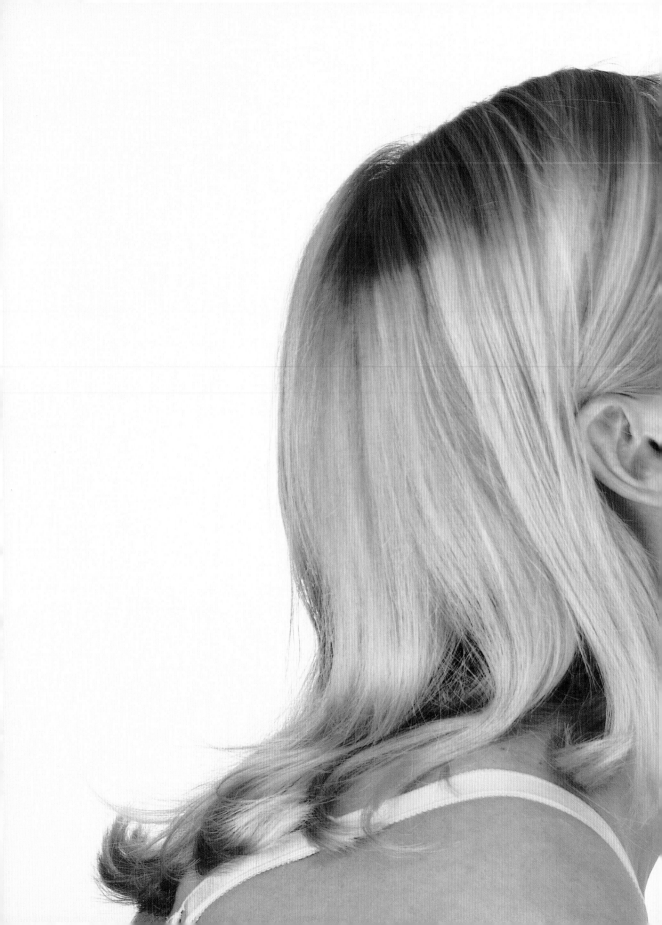

4 For the man in your life

(cunnilingus secrets you *need* your lover to know)

Personal story: **What do we want?**

What do women really want? That's the big question. I think what women don't realize is that men are really very simple — we just want them to be happy. We're trying to be New Men and in touch with our feelings and all that, but still we get accused of being selfish and inconsiderate. And the worst is when we're in bed.

I'd always considered myself a good lover until I met Sarah. I was 27 at this point and I met her in a bar. I was immediately attracted to her: she was small and very pretty, with a huge smile. She approached me as I waited at the bar to be served, and I couldn't believe my luck. We talked until we got kicked out of the pub and I offered to walk her home.

When we got back to the house she was renting a room in, she pushed me up against the front door. She was sexy and forward — she told me to come in for a coffee, then added with a sly smile, "Not that I have any." We kissed all the way upstairs and we were both naked by the time we hit the bed. She was amazing that first night — she really took control and wouldn't let me do anything. She gave me the best blow job I've ever had, then climbed on top of me and screwed me really hard. A couple of times I tried to do things to her — to reciprocate, really — but she pushed me away, saying she liked to pleasure me.

I thought I'd really hit the jackpot. We saw each other every single night, but after a while I was getting a bit annoyed. Every time we did it she was in charge, grabbing my hands and putting them where she wanted them. I tried again to pleasure her — I've always loved going down on girls and I really wanted to give Sarah oral sex — but every time she said "No" or just moved me into a different position.

I tried to tell my friend Miles what was going on, but he couldn't understand. He thought I should be pleased that I'd met a woman who loved sex so much, and said that if I didn't want her, he'd happily step in. So I thought it was just me. That I was being too sensitive.

But soon it was a real issue. The more Sarah took control; the less confident I became. I was scared to make any moves on her to try new stuff because every time she moved my hands away, I felt rejected. I started to go off her blow jobs too, which is unusual for me! It was just all her way, all the time. She would often get carried away, and I felt like I wasn't really there — that she was just using my dick to get herself off.

Anyway, after a couple more weeks she broke up with me, because her ex had said he wanted them to get back together. She also admitted to me that I wasn't "aggressive" enough in bed for her, that she liked a man to "take the initiative." I thought, "What? I would have taken the initiative if you'd only let me!"

The next girl I met was Jennifer. We'd known each other at college and met up at a reunion thing. I was still a bit bruised from Sarah, but when Jen asked if she could come back to my place after the party, I thought I'd give it a shot! What a difference—unlike Sarah, Jen was very shy in bed. When we were kissing on the bed, she didn't make any signs that she wanted to go further. It was like I'd keep doing stuff, expecting her to eventually stop me. Only she didn't. We did it that night and then the next morning too. At first, it felt really weird. I was still a bit self-conscious after the Sarah experience, so I went really slowly. I found that I kept asking her, "Is this okay?" and "Do you like this?" I felt a bit stupid saying that, because I had Sarah's voice in the back of my mind saying men should be aggressive. But I couldn't help it—I was scared to get carried away in case Jen didn't like what I did.

The next few times we did it were the same until Jen eventually admitted to me one night that she thought I was fantastic in bed, and that I didn't have to ask before I did stuff. She said she'd never had so many orgasms in her life, but my constant questioning was putting her off. She told me to relax.

So I did. With Jen I learned to regain my confidence, and every time she moaned or came, I felt a bit better. I'm still worried, sometimes, that I should be more forceful, or less anxious— I wish I could be somewhere in the middle. I don't think girls realize what an impact they can have on a guy's self-esteem. After Sarah I was really low, I thought I'd never have good sex again. I was questioning everything. But Jen helped me feel a bit better. We've split up now and I'm single, but I'm still looking for Miss Right. When I meet her, I know the sex will be fantastic, and that I can relax and just go with the flow."

Nick, 32

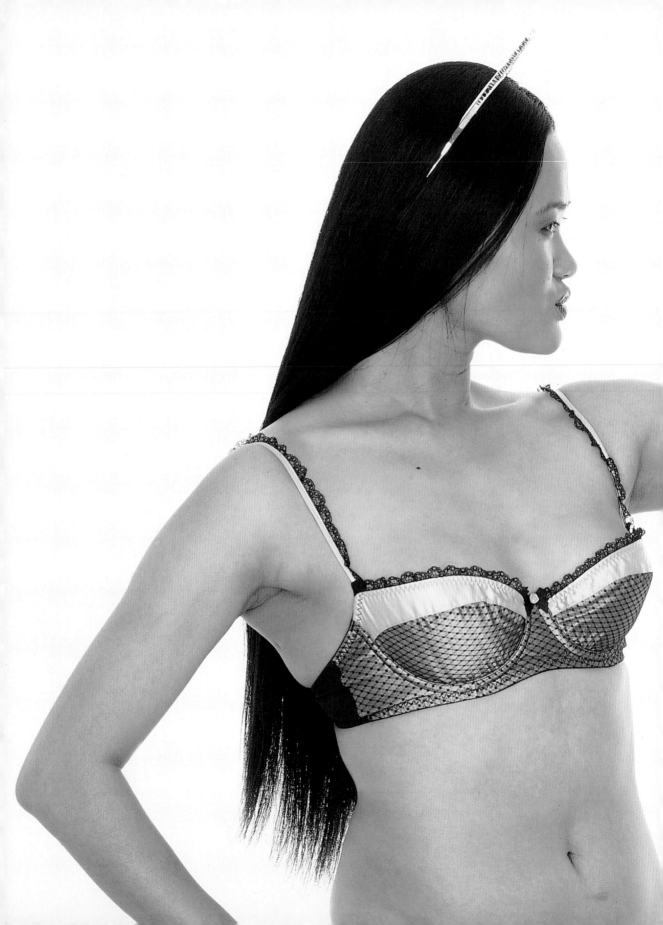

This chapter is for boys, so please pass it over to the man in your life. I'm going to tell him everything he's ever needed to know about pleasing you, from getting to know your private parts, to doing incredibly rude or brilliant things to them.

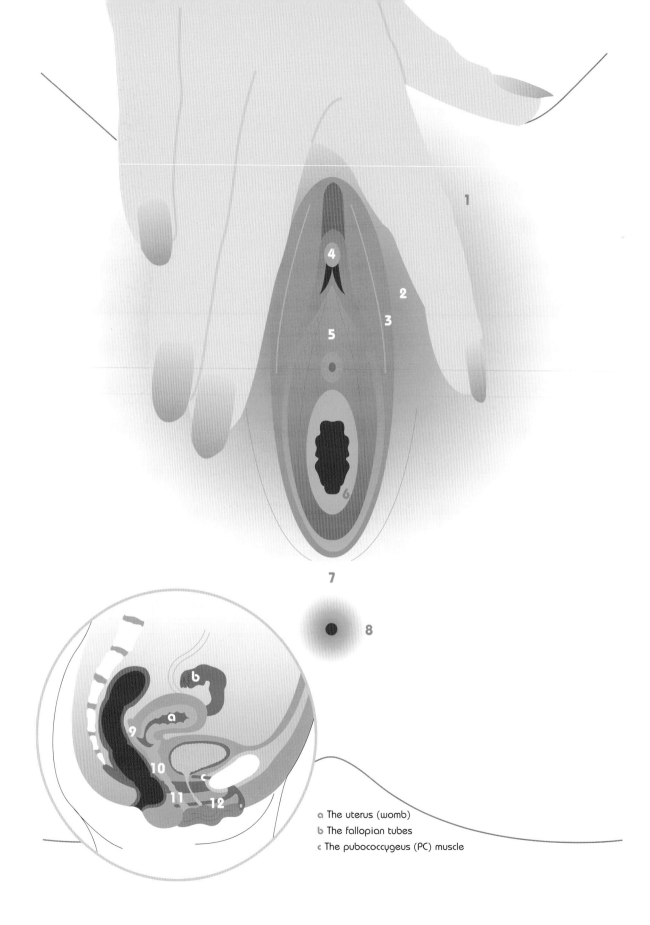

a The uterus (womb)
b The fallopian tubes
c The pubococcygeus (PC) muscle

Hello boys

First of all, don't take the fact that your partner has shoved this chapter under your nose as an insult of any kind. You're brilliant in bed, otherwise a) she wouldn't do it with you, and b) she wouldn't show you this bit because she'd know you wouldn't understand it.

This is a masterclass for men—a post-graduate course on how to perform cunnilingus so good, you'll be passed around all her friends as a kind of high-class call boy.

Know her private parts

1. The pubic mound (mons pubis)
This is a pad of fatty tissue that covers her pubic bone. The padding is there to protect you as you grind against it during sex.
Likes: Having its hairs stroked gently before oral sex (which is a great way to remove loose hairs, so you don't get them stuck in your teeth).
Dislikes: Having its hairs yanked or pulled or taken home as "trophies" (in case you were wondering).

2. The outer lips (labia majora)
These are usually covered in pubic hair, unless she shaves or waxes. They are made of erectile tissue (like the penis) and swell when the woman is aroused. They also share many of the same nerve endings as the clitoris, so they are very sensitive to the touch. Most men don't know that.

Likes: Being stroked and licked up and down.
Dislikes: Being touched too hard, being pulled.

3. The inner lips (labia minora)
These meet at the very top of the vagina to form a protective hood over the clitoris, in exactly the same way as your foreskin covers the head of your penis. These lips are hairless, and loaded with nerve endings that make them explosively sensitive. They are also erectile, so when she is very aroused they'll look puffier and darker in color. Note: the appearance of these inner lips varies greatly from woman to woman. Some are neatly tucked away, others hang below the outer lips. It makes no difference to their sensitivity, and smaller lips are just as responsive as bigger ones—albeit harder to find.
Likes: Soft licking, kissing, sucking. Sensitive to the tongue and fingers. Very, very, very.
Dislikes: Biting, nipping with the teeth (terrifying), being ignored.

4. The clitoris
Although the clitoris actually extends down the vagina lips, only the tip of it (known as the glans) is visible. It has a hood over it, like your foreskin, and is incredibly sensitive. Think of it like the head of your penis, and do unto it what you like having done to you. It's made of erectile tissue, which means it swells and hardens when aroused. Like penises, clitorises vary wildly in size. Some are big and, when

aroused, extend out from the vagina to a height of three-quarters of an inch. Bigger clits aren't more sensitive than smaller ones, just easier to find. Most women find direct clitoral stimulation too intense unless they are very aroused. Concentrate your early efforts around the clitoris, beside it or just below, gradually working inward as she gets more excited. It can get very sore from too much attention, just like the head of your penis.

Likes: Being gently stimulated, licked, sucked, tapped with fingertips.

Dislikes: Too much attention too soon, being bitten (hard), being rubbed when sore.

5. The urethral opening

This is where the urine comes from. Very sensitive to the touch. Some women can orgasm from having their urethral opening stimulated, which has led to it being called the "U spot."

Likes: Being licked and kissed.

Dislikes: Anything being poked into it. Eeek.

6. The vaginal opening

Ahh, the "gateway to paradise" as some pathetic creature once called it. This will usually look closed unless she is very aroused. Then the swelling of the lips will help to pull it open. The opening of the vagina and the first two or three inches inside it are the most sensitive areas. They are packed with nerve endings that will respond to your touch.

Likes: Being kissed, licked, fingered, having a tongue poked into it.

Dislikes: Sharp fingernails, having air blown inside (dangerous), being stretched too much by fists or sex toys.

7. The perineum

The flat stretch of skin between the vagina and the anus. Like yours, very sensitive to the touch.

Likes: Being massaged with flat fingertips, licking, kissing.

Dislikes: Being poked or jabbed.

8. The anus

This is the opening to the rectum and is usually closed. You should be familiar with it, having one yourself.

Likes: Varies from woman to woman, although licking and light fingering is usually a good bet.

Dislikes: Being fiddled with at all when she's paranoid about it not being clean.

9. The cervix

This is the entrance to the womb. It's tightly closed and usually covered with a thick mucus, to prevent infection spreading into the womb. During ovulation (the few days a month when the woman is fertile) this mucus changes consistency and becomes slightly thinner to help sperm pass through. You can often feel the cervix during sex—it feels like a piece of hard cartilage (sexy). Some women love having their cervix touched, either with fingers or a penis, and some hate it, so go carefully.

Likes: Varies from woman to woman.

Dislikes: Ditto.

10. The vagina

In its resting state, the vagina is about three inches long and flat (like a deflated balloon). However, during arousal it lengthens and opens out, to allow your penis access. It's lined with muscles and nerve endings (mainly in its bottom half), and glands that emit lubrication.

Likes: How long have you got? Responds well to being filled, which stimulates nerve endings.

Dislikes: Being stretched too much, or snagged with sharp fingernails.

11. The G-spot

For some women there is an area on the front vagina wall, two inches in and tucked behind the clitoris, that is incredibly, mind-blowingly sensitive to stimulation. It is known as the G-spot. Those who've found it say it is the size of a quarter and feels flatter and smoother than the rest of the vaginal wall. Stimulation of the G-spot can lead to female ejaculation, when a thin colorless liquid is released.

Likes: Being rubbed in circular motions with flat fingertips and/or a penis.

Dislikes: Prods, demented thrusts accompanied by shouts of, "Anything yet, darling?"

12. The crura

These are the internal wing-tips of the clitoris that run down inside the labia. Very sensitive.

Likes: Being rubbed, stroked and massaged through the labia.

Dislikes: Being ignored.

Now what?

Lightly running your fingertips over her tummy and into

her panties is never going to be a bad thing to do.

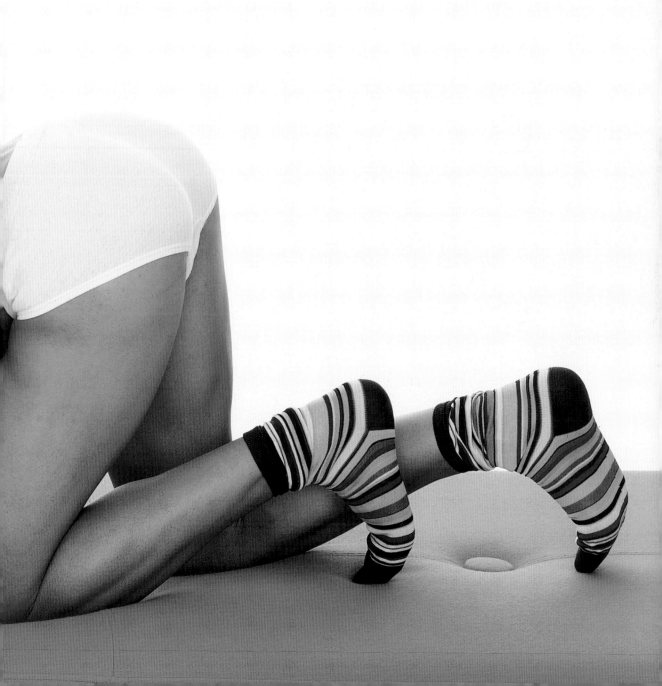

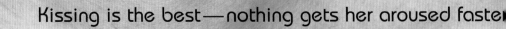
Kissing is the best—nothing gets her aroused faster

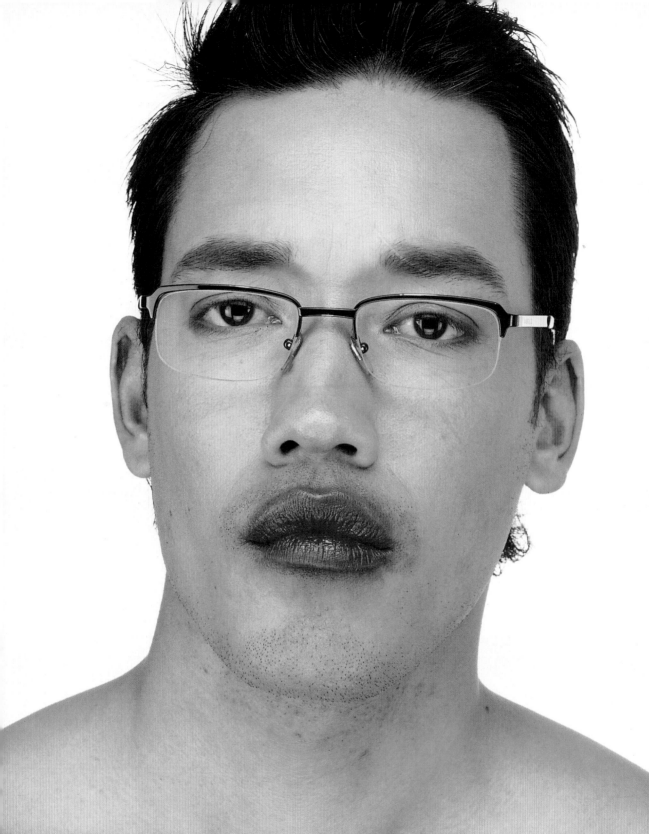

But it has to be good kissing, for a long time.

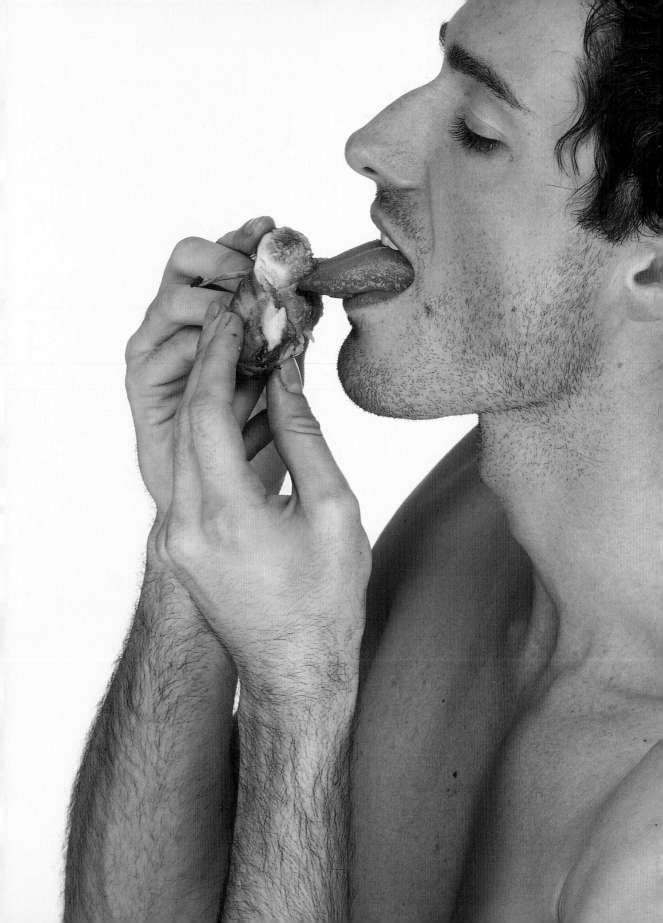

How to give perfect cunnilingus

So you've got your degree in gynecology, but what are you going to do with it? Here's how to put that knowledge to very good use.

Most women can't orgasm from intercourse alone, without any kind of added stimulation. Of course, some can—I don't want you to think everyone's been faking it all these years—but it's rare. The reason's simple: most sex doesn't stimulate the parts of our body that can make us come: the clitoris and sometimes the G-spot.

However, oral sex and hand jobs (fingering) are big-time orgasm givers. Oh yes. In surveys, oral sex comes out on top as the number one method, with fingering (or masturbation) slightly behind. So it's worth knowing how to get it right. Just as there is such a thing as a bad blow job, there is such a thing as bad cunnilingus. But not after you've read this.

Step 1: Arousal

Don't go rushing into her panties. It takes us a long time to become aroused and, before we are, it actually hurts to be played about with down there. Her being wet isn't a sign that she's ready for anything: we can be wet before you start, through normal secretions. The signs that she is genuinely aroused are the swelling of her labia, the erection of her clitoris, and the opening of her vagina. How do you cause these things to happen? Kissing and teasing.

Kissing is the best—nothing gets us aroused quicker. But it has to be good kissing, for a long time. Start by giving her slow kisses with your mouth closed, moving on to running your tongue over her bottom lip, finally working up to deeper French kisses. While you do, stroke the back of her neck with your hands. Like yours, our necks are incredibly sensitive and respond to everything. (While you're there, a string of kisses running from underneath our jaw around to the nape and back again wouldn't go amiss.)

Play with her breasts too. Yes, the nipples are sensitive but don't tweak them like you're tuning in to a radio station. A good tip is to gently stroke over them up and down with the palms of your hands. And stroke the underside of her breasts too—from under the nipple down to the crease where they join her body. So hot, your hands will melt. Kissing her nipples is a good bet—as is licking them from top to bottom with a flat, wet tongue. It gets annoying if you suck them too hard, so start by being gentle and trying a few playful nips with your teeth. Then gradually increase the intensity.

How long should you do this foreplay before you move south? For as long as possible, or at least until she starts squirming and opening her legs to show she wants you down there.

Step 2: Use your hands

Lightly running your fingertips over her tummy and down underneath the top of her panties is never going to be a bad thing to do. Tracing your fingers in her groin—the crease where the tops of her thighs join her pubic area—isn't either. Both are fab. What you shouldn't do is head straight for her vagina or clitoris. Keep touching her everywhere but, and you'll be working her up to such a state of excitement that whatever you do next will feel great. You want it to be an exquisite relief for her finally to be touched.

Step 3: Remove her panties

It's very sexy to be touched with your panties on, or through your panties. But then get them off. When the air hits the wetness of her vagina, it's heaven. So make sure she's lying down on her back, kneel between her legs and pull those panties off. Then kiss her, again, everywhere but her vagina. Kiss her inner thighs, trace your tongue along the gap between her outer lips, lick her perineum.

Step 4: Open her up

Place your hands on each inner thigh and use your thumbs to open her up. Stroke the tip of your tongue very lightly over her clitoris. Don't flick, just lick. It should be erect after all that foreplay. Make your mouth very wet (pretend you're chewing gum, to make more saliva), and place your lips over the entire clitoris.

Killer move no. 1: Lick the alphabet

This wasn't my idea, but it's awesome. With your thumbs still holding her lips open, use the tip of your tongue to start tracing the alphabet on her clitoris. A, B, C … What this gives her is varied stimulation—no lick is the same. (You could try any combination of letters or symbols but the alphabet is the easiest to remember.)

Killer move no. 2: Lick her up, lick her down

With a flat, wet tongue (not a sharp, pointy one), lick one stroke from her perineum right up to her clitoris. Repeat. Repeat. Mix this in with some more of those alphabet licks.

Killer move no. 3: Fingertips

Insert just the tip of your index finger inside her vagina. Just the very tip. Then move it around in circles, just inside. I can't tell you how pleased she'll be. All the best nerve endings are just there—except for the G-spot, which we'll get to in a minute.

Step 5: And finally

Combine licking with using your hands. These are all good techniques:

● Place your thumbs on either side of her clitoris and rub them in little circles while you lick over the head of it.
● Hold her lips open with the first two fingers of your left hand, while rubbing the sides of her clitoris around and around with the first two fingers of your right. Lick over the head of it.
● Lick inside her vagina while you use your

nose to rub her clitoris around and around.

● Suck the whole clitoris into your mouth and swirl your tongue all over it while you use your thumb to thrust inside her vagina.

● Hold the clitoris inside your mouth and shake your head from side to side, while thrusting with your thumb.

Step 6: Make her come

She might have come already, but if she hasn't —and you feel like your tongue's going to fall off if it takes much longer—you can switch to one of the following moves. But don't try these before she is very, very aroused—done too soon, they'll just hurt or annoy the tits off her.

The clitoris suck

Pull back the clitoris hood. With it fully exposed, put it in your mouth, give it a brief suck, then release. It feels incredible, but don't overdo it. Start with gentle sucks and build up.

The clitoris hold

Take her exposed clit into your mouth and gently suck on it, simultaneously flicking your tongue over and around it. This can be done lightly or aggressively according to what she likes, and combined with fingering.

The tongue tube

Roll your tongue into a tube around her clitoris. Slide it back-and-forth. In effect, your tongue is doing something similar to her vagina around your penis. Very, very hot.

Step 7: Start all over again

Women are different to men in so many ways— but the best difference (for us) is that we can have one orgasm directly after another. So after she's had one orgasm, there's no reason to stop. Probably the best method for giving her the second orgasm is through G-spot stimulation. It's not definite that your partner will either a) have a G-spot, or b) have a G-spot orgasm, but it's worth a go. In fact, she might orgasm as a result of your exploration, especially if you mix it up with clitoral stimulation too.

I hope you have handed this chapter over to your lover and he is taking heed. You will thank me some day soon for making him read this—that is when you have regained the energy to speak once you've been to heaven and back.

I hope you are enjoying your masterclass. Make sure you put all this knowledge to good use. Remember: don't go rushing into her panties, kissing will get her aroused quickly, as will playing with her breasts.

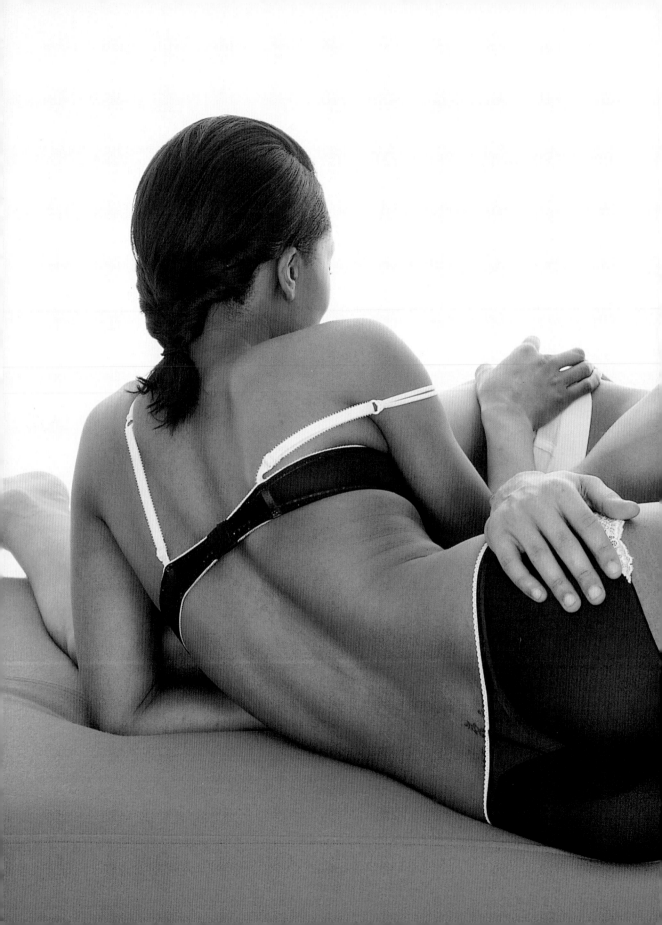

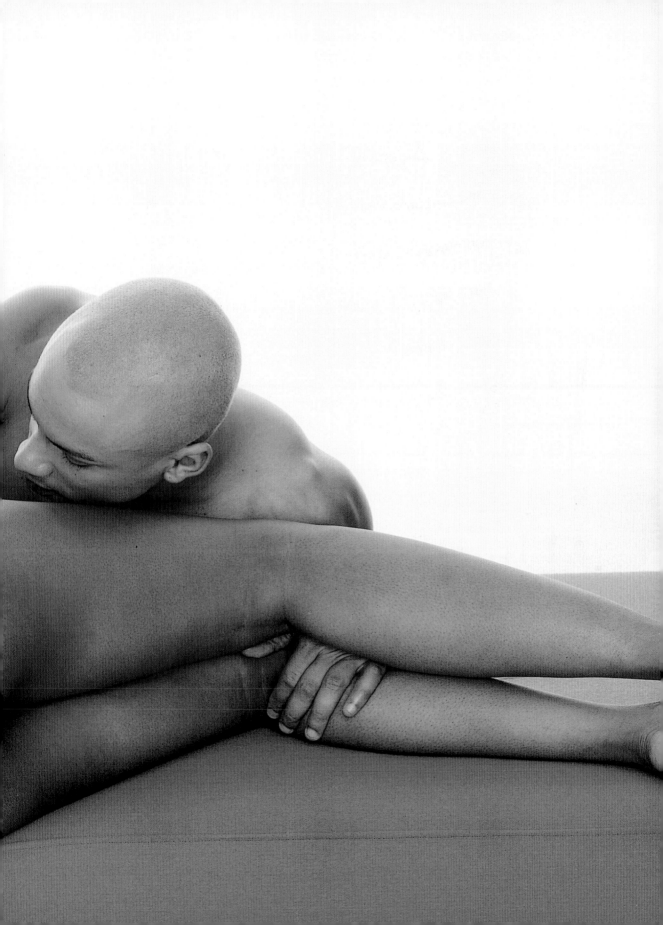

How to find her G-spot

Look at the diagram on page 96, and you'll see the G-spot on the vagina's front wall, i.e., the wall nearest her stomach. Think of it as under her clitoris you'll be on the right track.

Have your partner lie on her back. Kneel between her legs. With your hand facing palm up, insert two fingers inside her vagina, up to the second knuckle. Then curl the fingers towards you, in a kind of beckoning motion. You're now touching her front wall. With a bit of dexterous maneuvering, you may find a patch on that wall, about the size of a quarter, that feels different from the rest. That's her G-spot. (It might take a bit of time to find but don't worry—she won't mind a bit.)

When you've found the right area, press your two fingertips onto it gently, and then begin rotating them in a circular motion. The G-spot doesn't respond well to poking—you want to massage it with the pads of your fingers. Ask her what feels best.

How to give her a G-spot orgasm

Now, while one hand continues those circular massages, the other should get to work on her clitoris. Press either side of it and work in roundy-roundy motions; lift the hood with your fingers and swirl your tongue directly over the head; place a finger gently on the head and rub it as lightly as you can. Let her gasps guide you. With both hands working directly on her hot spots like this, she should orgasm. (It might

take a while—hang in there. Tutting impatiently and saying, "Look, the football game is on in a minute," isn't going to help anybody.)

Female ejaculation

Some women experience ejaculation from clitoral stimulation, but especially through G-spot stimulation. At the moment of orgasm, her vaginal walls will contract and she'll expel some clear liquid from her vagina. Some people say it's a lubricant, some say it's just fluid from her vaginal glands—but it's not urine. If you get covered in it, don't rush to the shower. Often if she does ejaculate, it's a sign that you have stimulated her to heavenly levels. An orgasm like that usually feels different to a clitoral climax—deeper, and as though her vaginal walls are "pushing out." It's amazing. She'll thank you. Oh yes. Expect a new car/TV/PS2 to be delivered within a matter of hours.

More techniques

Once you've mastered these techniques, you'll need some new tricks up your sleeve. So here are some other ways to show her you care.

Menthol mayhem

You know how sucking a cough drop makes your mouth feel all tingly? Well, it feels exactly the same on her vagina. So, suck one until it's a smooth, rounded shape—no sharp corners, please—then rub it over her clitoris and vagina. Make sure it's wet so it glides smoothly. Then blow on the area gently—the air will cool and heat her privates and it'll feel fab. If she's reluctant to let your Fisherman's Friends near her, you can just suck one then lick her with your mentholy saliva—not quite as good, but still good. Of course, mouthwash or toothpaste will have the same effect.

Rock her world

Some candy shops sell mint sticks that are about the same width as a penis. Suck one till it's smooth and rounded, then masturbate her with it. This feels awesome, and when you screw her afterwards, you'll see what I mean.

Exploring Uranus

The vagina shares a wall, on one side, with the rectum. Not only does this mean that sexual stimulation is possible from anal entry, it also means that a similar sensation can be achieved by stimulating the side of her vagina that shares nerves with her rectum. This is more or less the exact opposite, 180 degrees around, from the G-spot. Reach in and arch your finger to touch her G-spot, then rotate your hand to face the exact other direction and make a similar (but flatter) motion. This move rarely works well early on— you need to get her excited first. Press with the length of your finger, not the tip, stroking up and down. Mmmmm.

Around the world

Alternate G-spot stimulation with pressing on the other, anal, side. She'll feel G-spot stimulation, then anal stimulation, then G-spot, then anal … Remember to keep the moves specific to the side you're touching—when you're touching the G-spot, massage in little circular motions. Then switch to stroking your finger up and down the other wall. Got it? Try it now.

Labial hold

While holding the inner and outer labia together with your lips, run your tongue between them, one side at a time.

Tongue intercourse

The majority of her vaginal nerve endings are gathered around the opening and the first couple of inches inside her. Target them with your tongue by inserting it into her vagina. Techniques are fairly limited, due to the length of your tongue, but try moving your tongue in and out, as well as in circles around the inside of her and see if she doesn't appreciate it.

The flick

Spread her vaginal lips with your fingers. With your tongue pointed, gently flick your tongue around her clitoris. This drives some women wild, others find it to too intense. Start out gently if you aren't sure how she likes it.

Merry-go-round

Try tracing slow circles around the base of the clitoris with the tip of your tongue. If you vary the speed as you go, taking her through several waves of pleasure, but increasing speed all the time, you will not be disappointed with the results. Around and around and around you go, when she comes, you're sure to know.

Number's up

Use the tip of your tongue to trace a figure "8" around her clitoris. Don't be afraid to knock the clit around a little bit as your tongue darts first one way and then the other. She'll feel like you're coming at her from all sides. (This is a very good thing.) This requires some skill, a little tongue dexterity and stamina, but it's worth it.

Knocking on heaven's door

With your lips placed to each side of it, repeatedly "jam" your tongue downwards on to her clitoris. Don't worry if you don't hit it square-on every time, it'll still feel fabulous. Alternate with gentle sucks.

Lap of luxury

Lap across her clitoris and vagina with a flat, wet tongue. Pretend you are lapping a melting ice-cream cone. This feels particularly good when it's mixed in with more specific clitoris-moves, like the above.

Clitoral blow job

Begin by sucking slowly on the clitoris, as if you were giving it a tiny blow job. Gradually increase the intensity of the sucking, then begin to add a little flick from your tongue now and then. As she gets closer to orgasm, send her over the edge by continuously swirling your tongue around the tip of the clitoris while you suck the base of it.

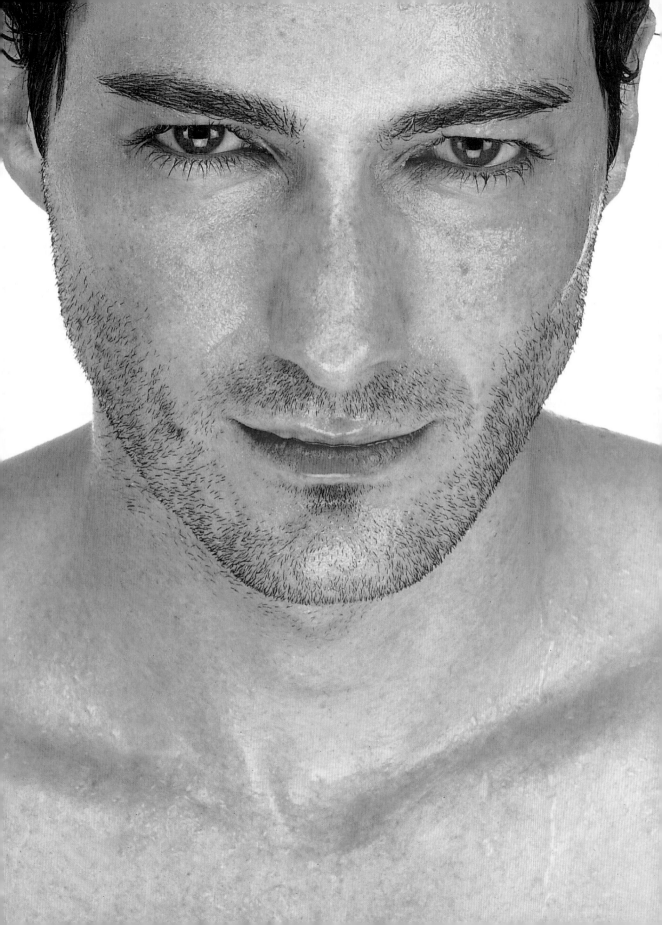

Q+A

■ **My girlfriend has had a lot more sexual partners than I have. I'm so worried about being good enough that it's affecting my performance. What should I do?**

● Just because she's had a lot of sexual partners doesn't mean they've been good lovers. If they had been, maybe she'd have stayed with them for longer. And she won't be thinking of you as inexperienced. Often people who have had fewer partners are better lovers because they have focused on someone they care about over a long period of time as opposed to having bad drunken sex with hundreds of strangers.

■ **I've noticed that my new girlfriend always gets particularly horny during her period. Is this normal?**

● There's a lot of research currently being done on just this subject. Biologically, women should feel horniest mid-month, when they're ready to conceive. But instead, lots of us feel sex-crazed either just before our periods start, or during them. The latest thinking is that it's down to hormones. Just before a woman starts bleeding, her estrogen levels dip, but her testosterone levels rise. That makes her feel sexier, as testosterone can affect the sex drive. (Testosterone might also explain her increased aggression just before her period. Tread carefully.)

Masturbate while you're giving her oral sex, and you'll keep tha

■ **I know that women love foreplay but I find that if I don't use my erection soon after I get it, it tends to go away and not come back. What can I do?**

● Well, don't panic, for a start. This happens to loads of guys. What you can do is stimulate yourself at the same time as you're stimulating her. Masturbate while you're giving her oral sex, and you'll keep that stiffy going strong. Or try 69s, so you both get in on the action. An easy way to do this is just to play with your penis with one hand. Don't worry about being "caught"—she'll be in the land of bliss, and won't notice a thing. If she does spot you, just tell her you were so turned on, you couldn't resist.

■ **Whenever I've slept with people in the past, they've been quite vocal during sex. The girl I've just started seeing is very quiet. She seems to be enjoying herself, though. Should I be worried?**

● No, not if she seems to be enjoying it. Why look for things to worry about? She's just not one of the red-hot screamers you knew before. Maybe her first sexual experiences were in a shared house where she had to be quiet; maybe an ex told her to shut up; maybe she goes into herself and prefers the strong, silent orgasm. It's usually the men that stay silent during sex. I've had to hold mirrors over guys' mouths in the past to check if they're still alive.

tiffy going strong.

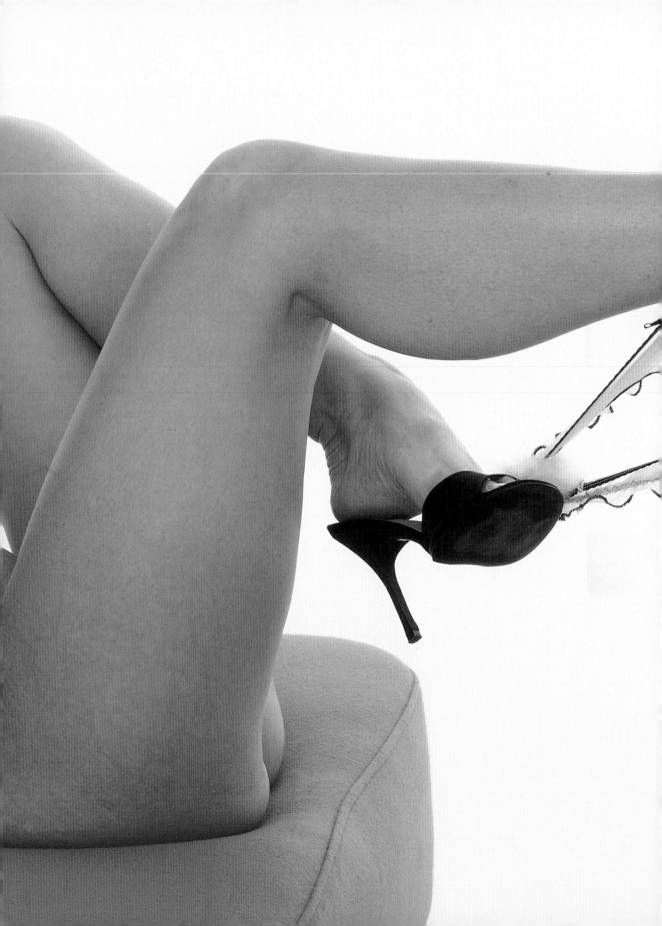

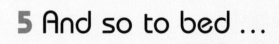

5 And so to bed ...

Personal story: **Position anxiety**

Every time I have sex, I can't help but feel that I'm the most boring lover in the world. Even though my partner seems happy—delighted, even, with our sex life, I can't lose the feeling that I'm really boring in bed.

I blame the movies. When you watch sex scenes in movies, do they ever do it like you do it? Never. It's always exotic and adventurous. They kiss, then—bam—she's on top, he's on top, the wardrobe is on top … They shift positions more often than a fidgety contortionist, racking up more variations in five minutes than I will in a lifetime.

The problem is, I only like sex when it's a bit familiar. I like the four basic positions: missionary, me on top, scissors and doggy style. I don't actually like anything else. Call me dull but I like my sex when it's easy, predictable and (most of all) comfy. I've read sex books before when they advised you to try all manner of moves. The wheelbarrow position for example, I mean, what's with that? Why on earth would being held over the carpet, head first, be in any way sexy? It's scary. I tried it once and all I could think was "Don't drop me…please, please don't drop me." He was like, "Are you getting there?" and I just wanted to scream, "Put me down, you maniac!"

Am I dull? I really don't know anymore. I've tried to broach the subject of positions with my friends but I feel like there's a veiled wall of secrecy. I can feel them looking at me in a weird way when I talk about it, and I'm afraid the look means, "God, she's hopeless in the sack." The only person I can really talk to about this is my brother. He's great and says that, actually, men hate all the fussy, changing-position stuff too. He says that basic nooky is the best for guys. I'm learning to believe him but I'd still like to know a few more killer moves to really surprise my man with.

Jane, 24

Sex tips

There's a joke about an old married couple that sums up the worst mistake women can make in bed. The husband comes into the bedroom stark naked. "Why aren't you dressed?" asks his wife. "Because I want to make love," he replies. "Over my dead body!" she retorts. "Of course," he answers, "that's the way we always do it."

If you want to be fabulous in bed, keep moving. Don't lie there passively. Be feisty; shake your booty. In the missionary position, raise your hips up to meet every thrust (or, for a sexy treat, ask him to stop moving and thrust your hips up to him). Use your PC muscles to squeeze and caress his penis. Scratch his back, bite his shoulder, gaze into his eyes and, if you like what he's doing, tell him. When you're on top, use your thighs to lift yourself far up off his penis and slowly slide back down. Even when he's taking you from behind, you shouldn't relax—thrust your hips backwards to meet every stroke, or grind them around and around.

Men need friction and depth to have great sex, so even if you're switching positions often, remember to include at least one that gives him a really deep ride. Women need a lot of clitoral stimulation to get off, so don't be afraid to masturbate yourself as you screw. He'll love watching you. Stroke your breasts too, lick your thumb and rub your nipples. Grab his buttocks and push him into you as deep as he can go. Do whatever you can to show him that you're enjoying yourself every bit as much as he is and he'll think you're a fabulous lover.

Of course, great sex is about both of you having a good time. The following list of positions includes tips for helping both of you climax, and sexy variations on every theme.

Let's go through them one by one. (Pretty much like you do with a new partner before you settle down to a routine of missionary, woman on top and the arms crossed, not-until-you-do-the-dishes position.)

Man on top positions

Missionary

The woman lies on her back, the man lies on top and penetrates her. Usually, he lies between her legs, which she then wraps around his waist or neck, depending on how much she ate for her supper.

You like it because: It's relaxing.

He likes it because: He's in control, deciding how deep to thrust and how hard.

Stimulates: Your emotions. This is the most romantic position, because you can easily kiss and caress each other and mutter sweet nothings. However, it's not the most physically stimulating position for either of you. In this position, your clitoris gets very little attention and your G-spot gets nuthin'. For the man it's better, but not much. His view is restricted (remember, men are all about visuals) and he can't see your gorgeous boobs bouncing around. But worry not, we have ways of sexing it up …

Make it orgasmic, for you: Stimulate your clitoris with your fingers. This is a great way to achieve orgasm in this position. If you're embarrassed, he can stimulate you with his fingers. Another good tip is to place pillows underneath your bum. This raises your hips so that he hits your G-spot with each thrust. (See Chapter 6 for more details on your G-spot.)

Make it orgasmic, for him: Raise your legs as high as possible. He can either hold both your ankles in front of his face (which is awesome), or you can hook them around his neck. The first improves his view and he can watch himself thrusting, and both positions alter the angle of your vagina so it feels tighter and more stimulating. This position also feels hotter for him, as it's more like hot movie sex.

Va-va-voom variations: Instead of him lying between your legs, you can lie in between his. Keep your thighs close together, so he thrusts between them into your vagina. This makes it feel hotter and tighter for him, and it stimulates your clitoris by putting more pressure on your pubic bone. Or, perform the normal missionary but have your head hanging over the edge of the bed. This forces more blood into your brain and women who've had orgasms in this position say they're ultrastrong. Alternatively, he can kneel up, which gives you G-spot stimulation and allows him or you to get at your clitoris.

Coital Alignment Technique

A version of the missionary invented by a psychotherapist and designed to help you climax. I want to see him get a Nobel Prize. Start off in the missionary position, with your man on top and inside you. He pulls out slightly, and positions his body so he is further up than normal. Rest your feet on his calves. His penis isn't deep inside you—the head is inside, but the shaft is outside, pressing on your clitoris. The movements are different too. No thrusting. He presses his pelvis down onto yours and rolls his hips. You rock up and down, ensuring your clitoris is stimulated at all times.

You like it because: His penis rubs against your clitoris, sending you to Happyland.

He likes it because: It's a slow, satisfying screw, and will probably make both of you orgasm.

Stimulates: Your clitoris, the shaft of his penis.

Make it orgasmic for you: Just make sure that he is rubbing your clitoris with every rolling move he makes, and you'll get there.

Make it orgasmic for him: Use your PC muscles to squeeze him, keeping him gripped tightly.

Va-va-voom variations: Doesn't need any, but after you've come, he can go back to thrusting, which should make him orgasm too.

Half-missionary

I call this the half-missionary because he's not between both of your legs. You lie on your back and raise your hips slightly. He then kneels on the bed at a slight angle to your body, one leg on either side of your left leg, and raises your right leg with his left hand. You keep your left leg flat down. He enters you at a slight angle, so his chest is behind that raised right leg.

You like it because: It reaches the parts that don't often get attention—his penis hits the side walls of your vagina.

He likes it because: Deep penetration (because your leg is raised), and he can last a long time.

Stimulates: Not great for hitting your G-spot, but you can manually stimulate your clitoris. He'll find it stimulates his shaft and glans in a new, rather lovely kinda way.

Make it orgasmic for you: Rub your clitoris and keep your leg raised high to keep him in deep.

Make it orgasmic for him: Hold his bum and really push him into you. A lot of men come when their buttocks are grabbed during sex.

Va-va-voom variations: Twist onto your left side, moving your right leg back over his body, and let him take you from behind while your knees are drawn up to your chest. Very hot.

▍Ultimo

A man-on-top position that some call "better than sex." Start by lying on your back. Your man kneels in-between your legs, grabs your calves and hooks them over his forearms. He is now supporting the weight of your legs and should pull your hips up off the bed. Now insert him into you. As you make love, he pulls you towards him by raising your legs. A great one for both of you, as he can see your whole body move (and watch himself penetrating you), and you get almost constant G-spot stimulation. Scorchio!

You like it because: Deep penetration and his penis rubs against your G-spot.

He likes it because: Deep penetration, a great view, and his testicles rub against your bum.

Stimulates: Your G-spot. At this angle, his penis will be rubbing that front wall of yours. For him, the deep penetration means that every inch of his penis is stimulated.

Make it orgasmic for you: When he is deeply inside, rotate your hips so that his penis rubs against every inch of your vagina. Use your fingers to rub your clitoris.

Make it orgasmic for him: It's pretty much guaranteed as it is. But for added oomph, reach down and hold the base of his shaft, keeping his foreskin pulled back so that the head of his penis gets extra stimulation.

Va-va-voom variations: From here, he could push your hips up and forward so you end up with your bum high in the air. He can then screw you more forcefully—which is nice. If he gets tired, hook your feet over his shoulders to give his arms a rest.

At this angle, his penis will be rubbing that front wall of yours.

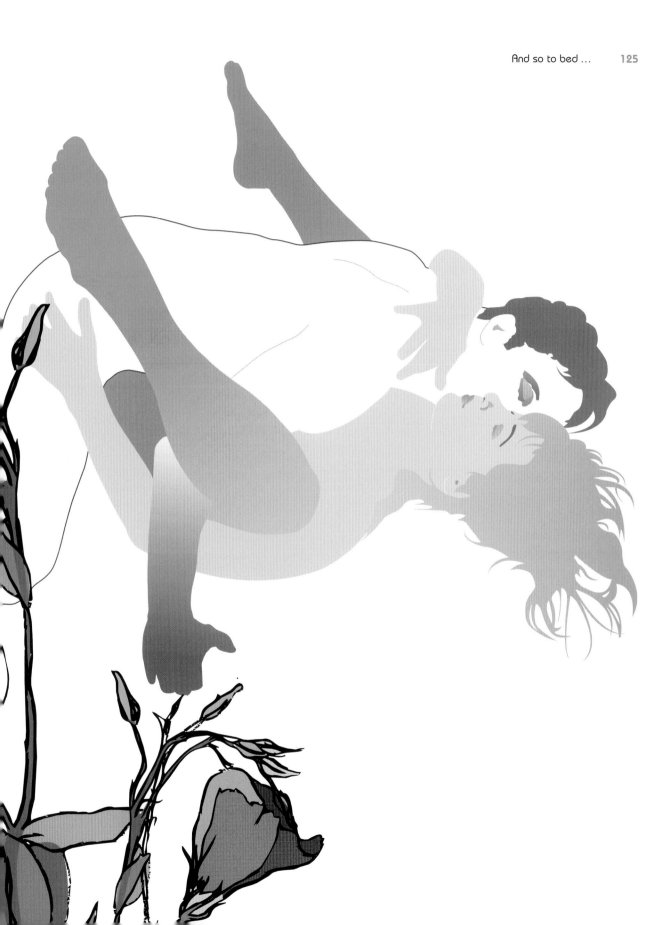

Woman on top positions

Inverted missionary

You lie on top of your man, so that your bodies are pressed against each other all the way down. His legs are together, yours are on top of his. You move yourself up and down his body.

You like it because: Your clitoris is pressed against his pubic bone, getting stimulated with every move you make.

He likes it because: You are very close together, he can feel your breasts on his chest. Plus he can usually last a long time this way as the penetration is relatively shallow.

Stimulates: Your clitoris.

Make it orgasmic for you: Grind your hips so that you're really rubbing your clitoris against his body.

Make it orgasmic for him: After you've come, lift your chest up, lean your weight on your hands, and thrust against him more forcefully. This will give him deeper penetration.

Va-va-voom variations: Keep your legs together, and get him to move his apart slightly. This will make it a tighter fit, and give every inch of his penis a blissful ride. Lift your hips off him slightly and, with your butt in the air, make rapid downward thrusts. Alternate them with slow grinding rotations.

▌The X

Start off on top of him, your legs on either side of his hips, his penis deep inside you. Then lean backwards until your back is flat on the bed. You'll both be lying on your backs.

You like it because: You can use your PC muscles to "milk" his penis, gripping him in hard so he doesn't fall out.

He likes it because: His testicles can get rubbed and stroked by your butt cheeks. And if he raises his head up with a pillow, he can watch himself screw you.

Stimulates: It just feels good. It's not a majorly stimulating position for either of you, but it's sexy to both lift your hips and grind.

Make it orgasmic for you: Masturbate yourself with one hand, and use the other to grip the base of his penis and stroke his testicles.

Make it orgasmic for him: Both of the above.

Va-va-voom variations: Don't lie flat back on the bed—lean halfway back, and rest your weight on your elbows. With your legs hooked over his hips, you can "shuffle" towards his dick, lifting your hips to thrust against him.

If he raises his head up with a pillow,
he can watch himself screw you.

Female superiority

For this, the man lies on his back. The woman straddles him, and works herself up and down on his penis. She can either rest her knees on either side of his hips on the bed, or she can give him and her extra thrills by squatting over him, feet flat on the bed, and using her thigh muscles to bounce up and down.

You like it because: It's the original feminist movement—literally. You're in control here and the depth of penetration and the speed of each thrust is dictated by you.

He likes it because: Not only does he have the best view of your whole body, but he can watch your face as you orgasm. And best of all, he feels he's being "taken."

Stimulates: Ooh, everywhere for you. Especially good for your G-spot as the penis rubs against the front wall of your vagina. Shallow thrusts are particularly good (if you can control yourself), as they stimulate the lower half of your vagina, where all the nerve endings live. For clitoral stimulation, ask him to masturbate you. He can easily reach from there and, really, it's the least he could do. This isn't actually the most stimulating position for his penis (we'll get to those positions next) but the view and the fact that you're taking him for your own pleasure will more than make up for it.

Make it orgasmic for you: Kneel astride him and grind your hips around and around in a circular motion. This hits everything, and gives you fabulous G-spot action. Alternate with thrusts for added oomph.

Make it orgasmic for him: Squat over his penis and use your thighs to lower yourself up and down (easiest if you have a headboard you can hang on to). This gives him the friction he needs. If you can pause between thrusts and leave his penis just inside your vagina, teasing him before you lower yourself back down— ooooh. Also, if you play with your breasts he'll think he's died and gone to heaven.

Va-va-voom variations: Face backwards, towards his feet. He'll love that as he can see your delicious butt, and because you can lean forward and lick his toes. Tingle-tastic. Just before he comes, pull gently on his big toe. Men say this can give them longer, stronger orgasms. If you're feeling especially athletic, try giving him an "Around the World," where you rotate yourself around on his penis. Tricky to master but proposal-inducingly good if you do. For you, a sexy variation is to lean forward, resting the palms of your hands on his chest, and work your hips forward and back. It rubs his penis directly against that extra-sensitive front wall of your vagina. Bliss.

Rear-entry positions

Doggy-style

A male favorite. The woman kneels or lies face-down and is penetrated from behind. The vagina is shortened, so he feels bigger. Great for pregnant women as there's no weight on the stomach if she rests on her hands.

You like it because: You can fantasize that it's Johnny Depp back there.

He likes it because: He can fantasize that you're Salma Hayek. And watch his penis thrusting into you—his favorite view in the world.

Stimulates: A G-spot winner—he hits the front wall; the extra depth gets him off. From behind he can thrust in deeply. Shout if it hurts.

Make it orgasmic for you: Play with your breasts—when they're hanging down (as they are in this position) they're extra sensitive. Rub your clitoris or hold your labia together as he thrusts between them—very hot for both of you.

Make it orgasmic for him: Reach between his legs to stroke his balls. Like your boobs, they're more sensitive when swingin' free. Be warned—he won't last long with that kind of attention.

Va-va-voom variations: Pillows under your hips alter the angle for deeper penetration. Or he sits back on his heels, pulling you onto his lap: G-spot stimulation, and added depth for him.

Wheelbarrow

Does anybody really ever do this? It's very hard work. However, there are gains to be made—mainly G-spot stimulation and deep penetration—so if you've never tried it, try it now. Just once. Just so you can say you have. Start by standing up, then bending forward and touching your toes. Your man stands behind you, inserts his penis, then hooks a hand under each of your thighs. You lift your feet off the floor, rest your whole weight on your hands and he screws you.

You like it because: Very deep penetration, lovely G-spot action and a head-rush.

He likes it because: It's a classic porn-film move, giving him loads of penetration and a great view.

Stimulates: Your G-spot, his penis.

Make it orgasmic for you: Just enjoy the ride.

Make it orgasmic for him: Squeeze and release your PC muscles against his penis. And try not to fall over.

Va-va-voom variations: Slightly less exotic but much easier is just to stay in your original toe-touching position and do it like that. It feels really good. He won't last very long with all the excitement, as it'll give him such a deep, satisfying screw.

Side-by-side positions

Spoons

The woman lies on her side, the man lies behind her. Popular among the pregnant as no weight is on the stomach. Also good for people who are tired and fancy a relaxing, soothing screw. Not very deep penetration but lovely. The best position for anal sex if it's the first time.

You like it because: It feels more romantic than doggy-style. He can play with your privates.

He likes it because: Well, it makes a change.

Stimulates: Your G-spot. Penetration is quite shallow. But he can stroke your butt and you can reach back and play with his testicles.

Make it orgasmic for you: Stimulate your clitoris manually. Rub yourself up the right way. Bringing your knees up to your chest deepens penetration; keeping them down ensures his penis is in that sensitive lower vagina.

Make it orgasmic for him: Reach around and hold the base of his penis. What this will do is keep his foreskin (if he has one) pulled back, so he feels more with every thrust. If he's circumcised, still do this—he'll enjoy the feeling of your hands more than he can ever express.

Va-va-voom variations: Bring your top knee up leaving the other straight and have him enter you at more of a right angle—deep penetration.

▌The hands-free

The man lies on his side, the woman on her back at a right angle to him with her knees bent over his hip. Again good for people who are tired and fancy a relaxing screw; but no good if you want to kiss—you can't reach.

You like it because: Everybody's hands are free to roam where they will.

He likes it because: The workload is shared equally.

Stimulates: Generally. And the penetration is deep for such a relaxed position.

Make it orgasmic for you: Once again, stimulate your clitoris manually—preferably while he plays with your breasts. And alternate between being still and moving.

Make it orgasmic for him: Thrust him further into you by leaning forward, reaching between your legs and pulling him towards you, or by propping yourself up on your elbows, arching your back and thrusting towards him.

Va-va-voom variations: With deftness, this can be turned into spoons or doggy-style. Swivel your legs around and over his so that he's behind you, or swivel one leg the other way, while you get him to lie on his back, and you're on top, straddling him.

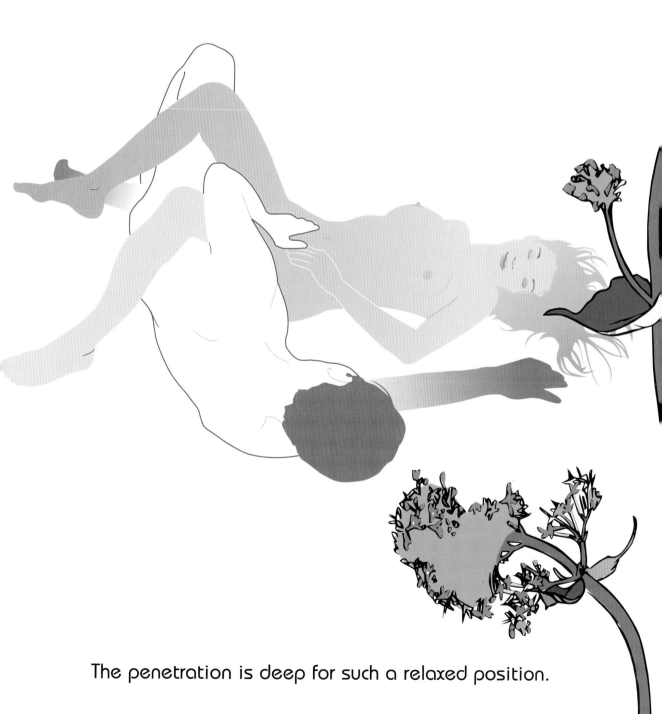

The penetration is deep for such a relaxed position.

Sitting positions

You on top of him, facing him

You've probably done this before, with great success. Very good for a quickie. He sits with his thighs together, you hop aboard and raise yourself up and down. Good for your G-spot, and gives him loads of penetration, especially if you rest your weight on your feet rather than your knees, so you can really bounce up and down.

Try this: On the sofa, armchair, on the backseat of your car, airplane restroom, train compartment, during a picnic.

▌You sitting on top, facing away

Easiest if he is sitting on a low chair, so you can rest most of your weight on your feet. Good for deep penetration, especially if you lean forward and touch the floor. Better with older men— young guys' erections are so tight to their tummy, that they find it hard to bend them downwards. You can also vary things by having him sit on the floor, while you crouch over him.

Try this: On the stairs, in the car, airplane restroom, bathroom, train compartment, outside (if you are wearing a long skirt).

Him half-sitting on the bed, you straddling him

Like woman-on-top, but instead of lying down, he sits up. Very good for kissing and romantic face-stroking stuff. Also slightly better than normal woman-on-top as it hits your G-spot more. You can reverse this too, so you face away from him. Less romantic but easier for you to stimulate your clitoris and his testicles.

Try this: Any time, any place, anywhere.

Him half-sitting/kneeling on the bed, you lying back, him holding your hips

Oooh, this is good. He pulls you onto his dick with every thrust. Start in the above position then lower yourself back down onto the bed.

Try this: As above.

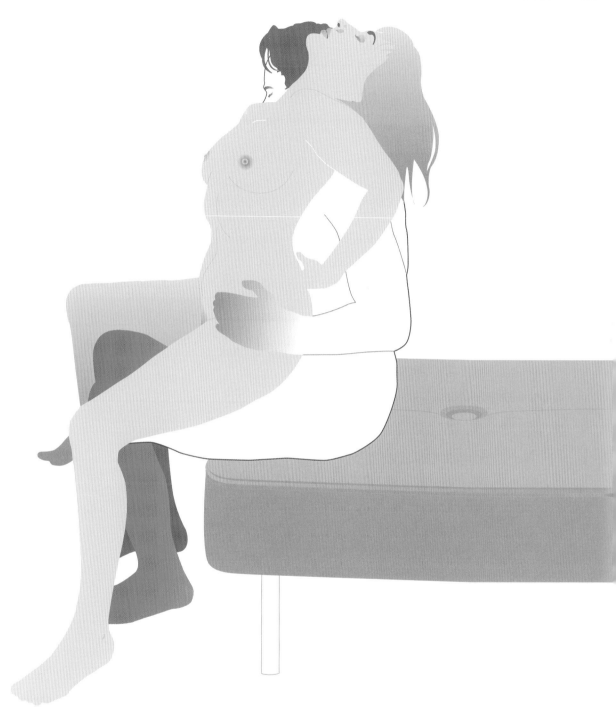

Good for deep penetration, especially if you lean forward
and touch the floor.

Standing positions

▍Both standing up, him entering you from behind

You have to be almost the same height for this to work. If you're taller than he is, you'll have to bend your knees to be low enough for him to enter you. If he's too tall, he'll have to crouch. You can get the heights right if one of you stands on a box or a stepladder. Great for quickies where you might get caught.

Try this: On your way home from a party; before he leaves for work in the morning; in the shower (use lots of lube as water can dry you out); in an alleyway—like *9½ Weeks*.

Him standing, holding you in front of him

This is what's known as a "knee-trembler." Can be great if he's strong enough to support your full weight the whole time. Can be easier if he's standing in front of something you can rest your knees on, like a kitchen counter or a desk.

Try this: In the kitchen, his office, your office.

Him standing, holding you underneath your thighs, you facing away from him

Unless you weigh less than a rice cake he'll never be able to keep this up. Great penetration—he can raise you up and down onto his erection. Popular in porn films, rare in real life.

Try this: In front of a bed in case he has to drop you suddenly when his arms go into spasm.

You lying on your back, him standing in front of you

Perfect in the kitchen on the counter. He has a great view from here, and some men say they like it because they can smell more of your "scent." Keep your back straight—this is easiest if you hook your feet over his shoulders. Very, very good for G-spot stimulation.

Try this: In the kitchen, on your desk, on the bed (with him kneeling instead of standing).

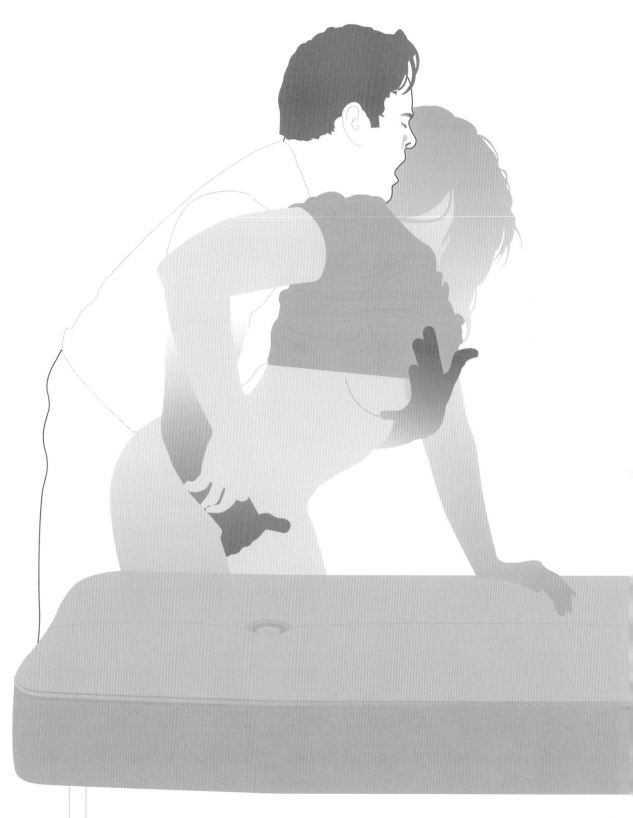

A tip to send him over the edge: When you've had a wonderful night with your man and you've come at least once and now you are exhausted but he's still going strong, wet your finger and reach round to give him a light anal tickle.

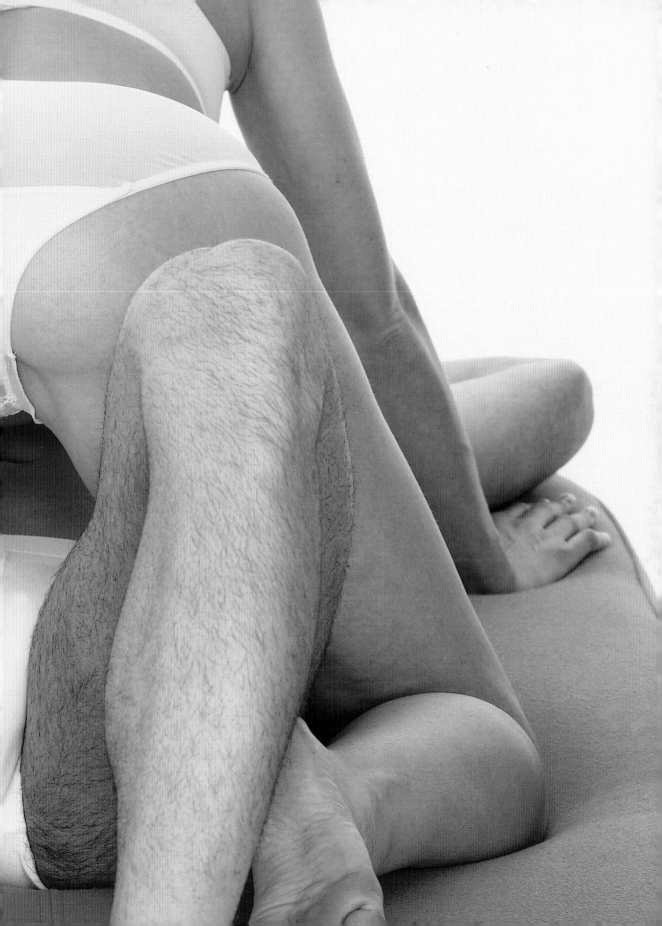

Anal sex

Are you ready for the last taboo? Anal sex is the "dirtiest" act most of us can imagine. It's rude, it's naughty and it's rare. So, of course, it's a very popular male fantasy. If you've tried anal sex before, I'd bet my house that it was on the suggestion of a boyfriend. Few women volunteer for this—usually, the man nags until she agrees out of curiosity or the desire to shut him up.

However, after that scary first time, many women enjoy anal sex. Apart from the mental reasons (it is "dirty" and dangerous and exciting), physically it can feel good. The anus and the vagina are very close together after all, and share some nerve endings. During anal sex you can feel the penis rubbing against the vagina, which is sexy, and you can easily masturbate or use a vibrator to gain added vaginal stimulation.

Men like it for the obvious reason—friction. The anus is very tight and small, and gives the penis about the most intense squeeze it can get. I also suspect there's an air of domination about it, especially if he's had to persuade you to give in to his request. But that's no reason to do so—if the idea makes you uncomfortable, you don't have to agree. In fact, there's a very easy way to turn down his suggestion for anal sex, which won't hurt his feelings or leave you looking like a prude: tell him his penis is simply too big. You'd love to but he's too much of a man, it'd be agony. He might be slightly saddened that he's not going to get any backdoor lovin', but he'll get over it.

Health and safety

We can't talk about anal sex without mentioning AIDS. If you're going to try it and haven't both received a clear HIV test, please use a condom. In fact, use a specially thick one designed for anal sex. The membranes in the anus are very delicate and can tear easily, which increases the risk of a virus passing between you. A condom won't lessen his sensations or yours—your anus is so tight he'll get plenty of friction. The other crucial health tip is do not insert anything into your vagina after it's been in your anus without washing it first. There's loads of bacteria living up your butt—don't let 'em spread to your vagina, okay? Promise me? Yes? Then you're ready to begin.

Anal sex for the first time

Are you sitting comfortably? You won't be in a minute. (I'm kidding.) The most important tip for anal sex is lubrication. Lots of it. Unlike the vagina, the anus isn't naturally lubricated so bring your own. I recommend Astroglide or K-Y Jelly (saliva dries too quickly).

Start by kissing and caressing. Have him go down on you. While he's there, he can start rubbing your anus with a fingertip. Tell him to take it slow, you have to get used to this. When you're aroused, he can insert just the tip of his little finger—well lubricated—into your anus. When you're ready, he can push it in a little deeper, up to the second knuckle.

Will there be poo?

No, there won't. Feces only enter the lower half of the butt just before you go to the bathroom. The rest of the time it's miles up inside your bowel. Have a bath beforehand, but otherwise don't worry.

The next step is for him to insert two fingers into you—probably his index finger and middle finger. Then try this call-girl tip: with two fingers inside your anus, he can pour lubricant down the fingers so it goes directly inside you. Then you're ready to try penetration.

Don't try it doggy style the first time—it's too frightening. You can't control the depth of penetration and you'll never be able to relax enough to enjoy yourself. Instead, get into the spoons position. Lubricate his condom-wrapped penis and, reaching around behind you, guide it towards your anus. Let the head rest against the opening until you're ready, then gently—I said gently—guide it in. As soon as the head's inside, stop. Don't make any sudden moves. You have to adjust to the sensation of being penetrated in this way. Unless he's enormous, it won't hurt—but you'll still need an adjustment period. When you're breathing normally again, push back against his penis to slide more of it inside. Then you can start making love, with him pushing into you with slow, gentle strokes.

If you need more stimulation, he can rub your clitoris and insert fingers inside your vagina. He can also stimulate your G-spot (see the next chapter for details). Many women can come this way. After you've both finished he should hold the condom securely around the base of his penis and withdraw slowly.

Will my butt be affected?

No. It takes a lot of penetration before your anus is stretched or weakened.

Other anal sex positions

After that first time is, er, behind you, you can try other ways. The most common is doggy-style, but missionary works well too—he just inserts his penis into your anus rather than your vagina. This way you can still hold his penis to control the depth of penetration.

Anal sex for him

Almost every man greatly enjoys having his anus stimulated, by licking or gentle fingering. But some want to go further and have a dildo inserted up there. If your partner wants to try this, and it's okay with you, repeat the above directions but in reverse, i.e., you lie behind him so he can guide the well-lubricated dildo into his bottom. Then you can hold it and push it in. Tell him to say how he likes it, and to warn you when you're going too hard or fast. And don't try it when you're in a bad mood with him—the urge to shove it in eye-wateringly hard would probably be impossible to resist.

The male G-spot (the prostate gland) is located up inside his butt. So, obviously, it's going to like some gentle stimulation. Start by rubbing his anus with a lubricated finger. If he likes it you can go a little deeper.

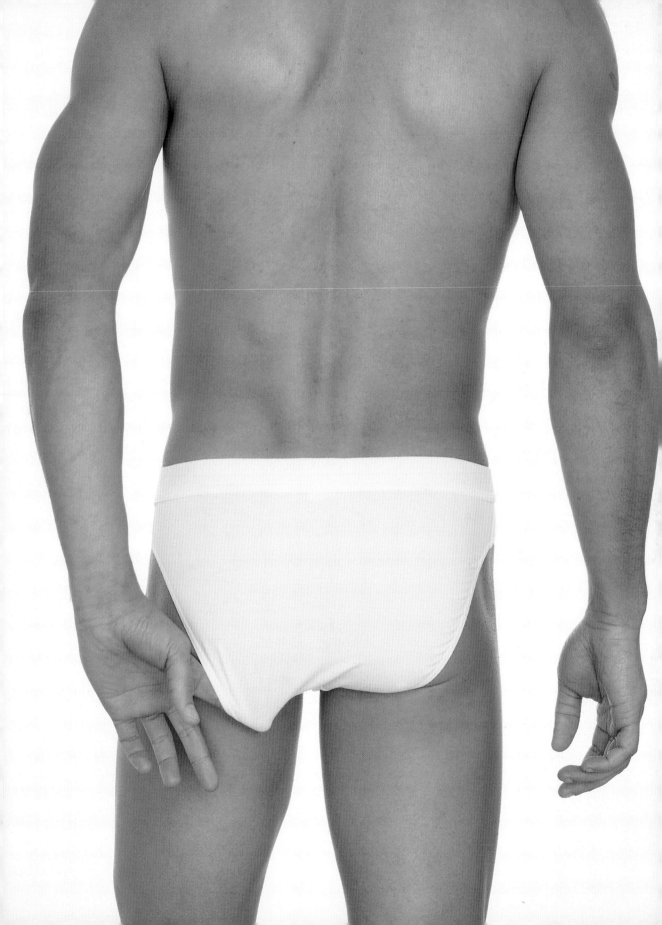

Don't get fantasies and fetishes mixed up. Fantasies are purely mental pictures that arouse you. Fetishes are specific sexual acts that turn you on.

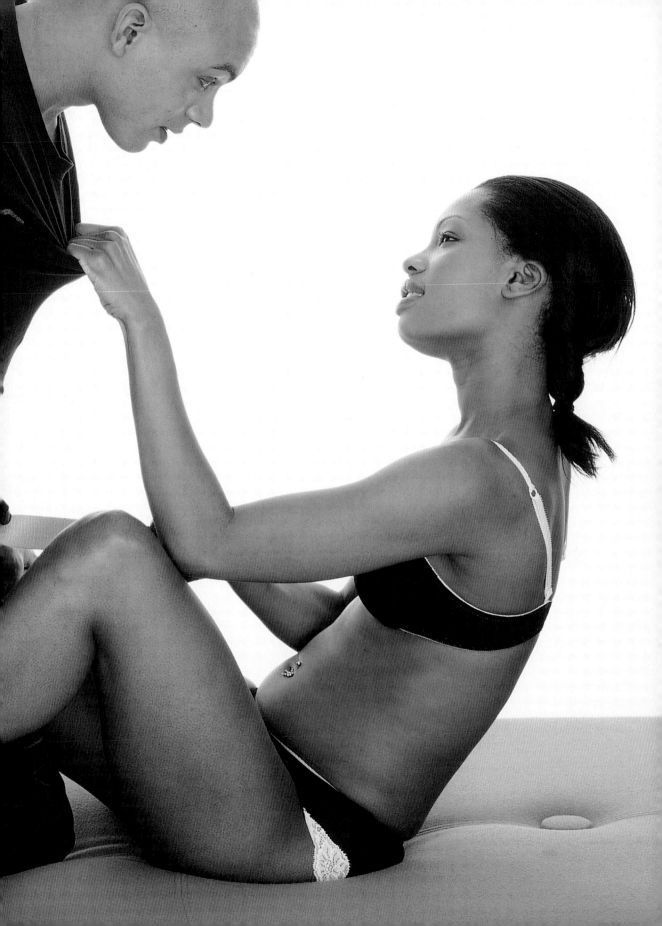

Fantasies

Never feel embarrassed about the fantasies you enjoy. I mean, never. And don't get into a panic attack because you love to dream about men with three dicks, or being "forced" to have sex with a stranger. These aren't deep-seated psychological messages being sent from your brain. They're just sexy ideas that you enjoy thinking about.

All of us have weird fantasies from time to time, or all the time. I can't even begin to tell you some of the nonsense that's gone through my head during sex, or when I'm alone in my bedroom. If I told anyone, I'm sure they'd lock me up and force-feed me sedatives for the rest of my life. But it doesn't mean anything—they're just sexy ideas that pop into my brain.

If you get turned on by thinking of lesbian sex, it doesn't mean you're gay. If you find the idea of doing it with your dog arousing, it doesn't mean you're going to end up on a bestiality charge. For some reason, we all get turned on by all kinds of nonsense. We're human. We're the only species that can achieve orgasm using mental stimulation and by god, is it ever fun!

The only time it does get tricky is when you want to act out your fantasies. Most of us never do, and I think that's a good idea. I know I sound like a bore saying that, but fantasies are like films—you can direct the whole thing in your mind. As soon as you bring them out into real life everything changes: you hate his boxer shorts, he gets his lines wrong, you get the giggles, the dog escapes and runs out of the room … It's never as good as it was in your mind.

Don't get fantasies and fetishes mixed up, either. Fantasies are purely mental pictures that arouse you. Fetishes are specific sexual acts that turn you on. If you find yourself having the same fantasy—say, bondage—over and over, it might be a fetish. But if you definitely cannot orgasm without fantasizing about that specific act, then it's definite. Look it up on the internet—you'll probably be surprised how many other people share your fetish, and you might look into meeting up with like-minded souls. Just be very careful and don't ever meet anyone without others knowing where you're going, and how to contact you.

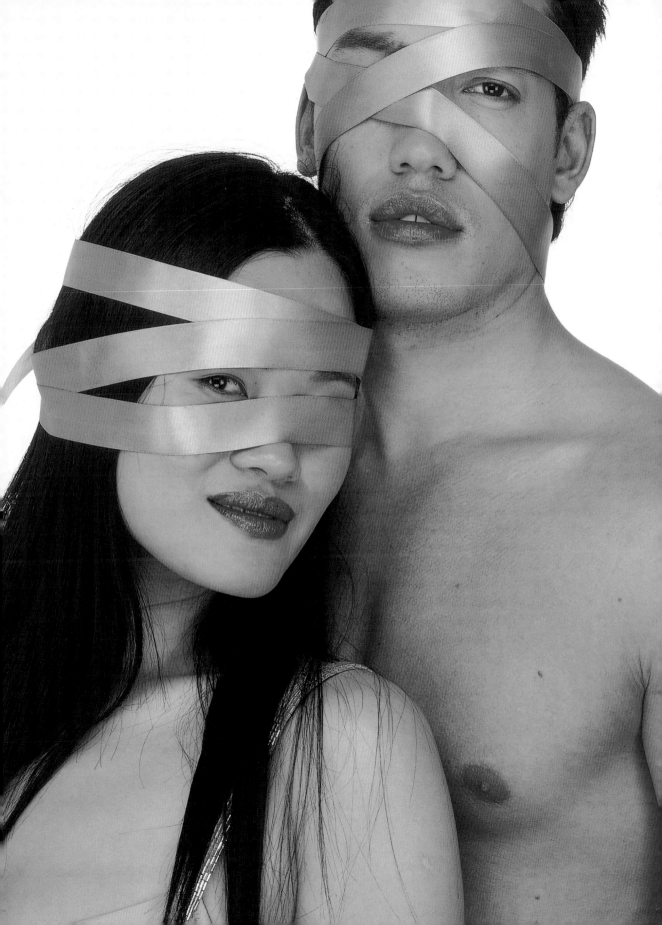

Q+A

■ I love sex with my boyfriend but he always comes very quickly. How can I prolong the pleasure?

■ I've had three children. Since the birth of the youngest, my husband has mentioned that my vagina isn't as tight as it was. He says it's harder for him to maintain his erection inside me. Help!

● Probably the easiest way is to masturbate him first, or give him a blow job. After he has come the first time, then have sex with him. He'll be desensitized and last longer second time around. Another way is to try some of the positions listed before that don't give him too much stimulation—try spoons or you on top. His penis won't be getting as much stimulation as it does in missionary or doggy positions, and you should find he keeps going longer. Or you can buy desensitizing oils which slightly numb the head of his penis and help him go longer. Finally, if he's not already, have him wear a condom. As well as protecting you from everything, it'll dampen the feelings and help him last the distance. Good luck.

● During natural childbirth the walls of the vagina have to stretch considerably. After three kids, I'd imagine your vagina has been stretched quite a lot. Don't worry—it's not unfixable. The first thing to do is exercise your PC muscles (see p. 96). To find them, try to stop peeing midflow. Those muscles you have to clench and pull up are your PCs. Start clenching and unclenching them, as hard as you can, whenever you can; these are Kegel exercises. Aim to do sets of 20 clenches, three times a day. Try that and see if it works. But give it a good go—nothing will change in a week but after three months you should see dramatic results. Using those muscles you can grip and squeeze his penis. Another tip is to try doggy-style sex—the vagina feels much tighter.

Men like doggy-style because it gives them deep penetration

■ My boyfriend wants to have doggy-style sex with me, but I'm not enthusiastic. It seems really unromantic and impersonal.

■ I can't come just from intercourse. This isn't something that my friends and I talk about. Am I odd?

● Sigh. Can I rant? I'm sorry but whining like this really get on my nerves. Sex is sex. It's not meant to be romantic. It's meant to be sexy, exciting and fun. The romantic part happens before you have sex, and afterwards when he brings you tea and sleeps on the wet spot. Obviously, if you're worried that your boyfriend is unromantic and impersonal towards you the rest of the time, you have a problem. But really, good sex isn't all about face-stroking and whispering "I love you." Sometimes it's fast, furious and frantic. Men like doggy-style because it gives them deep penetration and a glorious view of your butt. Just because he can't see your face doesn't mean he doesn't love you. Don't do it if you're not happy to, but don't invent things to make you miserable.

● No. Most women can't come from intercourse alone. It doesn't give us enough stimulation on our clitoris to make us orgasm. We're badly designed—our clits are way up out of reach and never get stimulated by just the in-out bit of sex. Rub your clitoris as you screw (or ask him to), or try extending foreplay for as long as possible. When you're really, really excited—I mean, "Get that into me now!" excited—you might be able to come when he first thrusts into you. If not, simply masturbate as you make love. Lots of women do that and achieve blissful orgasms. (No, your partner won't mind. In fact, he'll probably find it sexy to watch.) Good positions for easy access to your clitoris are missionary, you-on-top and scissors. Just keep rubbing until you feel your orgasm building, then tell him, and you can come together.

nd a glorious view of your butt.

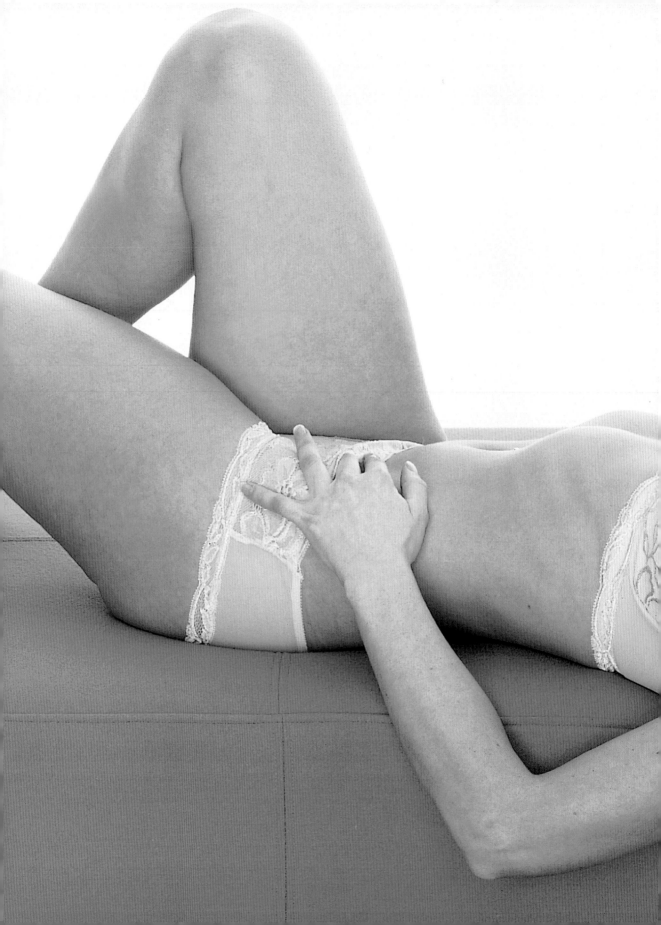

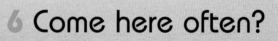

6 Come here often?

Personal story: What an orgasm feels like

I usually know before I have sex if I'm going to come. It's like my body is either ready for it or not. During the kissing stage, I usually become aware of a desire to be penetrated—it's like I just want my boyfriend inside me, right then. I have a dull ache down low in my stomach, which I know is me getting wet. If the man is a new partner, just kissing alone is enough to get me very excited; with a regular partner, it takes a bit longer.

When we start making love, that first thrust is fantastic. As we carry on, I start to masturbate my clitoris. It's usually erect by then, and I find that if I squeeze my fingers down on either side of it and press, that feels good. About a second before I actually come I feel a sharp heat all around my pelvis, then a tingly sensation in the lower half of my vagina. Then it's like a jolt: my back arches, I stop breathing for a split second, and I start contracting around his penis. It always feels to me like I'm really squeezing him, but some boyfriends haven't noticed it at all. While I'm actually contracting, I don't want any extra stimulation at all—if he keeps thrusting it puts me off a bit—and I stop rubbing my clitoris. It lasts about five seconds, then fades away.

Afterwards I really like him to keep thrusting, although my vagina feels quite big by then. I don't get the same friction any more as I'm so wet, and he has to go deep for me to feel anything. I know loads of women say that, with extra stimulation, they can have another orgasm immediately, but it takes me a while. However, if he keeps thrusting, and I start pressing down around my clitoris again, I can have another orgasm, and another, almost indefinitely. The second or third orgasm is usually better than the first, with longer contractions and more heat.

Julia, 23

Why and how do women orgasm?

Can you believe that scientists are still asking that question? It's not enough that women can have lovely orgasms through sex—the experts have to find out why we can. Oooh, men make me angry sometimes. But I suppose they have a point. Unlike male orgasm—where sperm are sent flying on their mission to make a baby—female orgasms don't appear to have an obvious reproductive function. You can still get pregnant even if you don't come. So why do we come?

Research suggests that it may be for one of two main reasons. The first is that it does help us get pregnant: during the female orgasm, the vaginal walls contract rhythmically, helping to push the semen up towards the cervix. The cervix itself also changes, dipping down during the climax, and "sipping" daintily at any sperm that's waiting there. That's one school of thought. The other is that our orgasm is a kind of reward. For us, sex can lead to pregnancy and having to look after a child until it's old enough to go kill its very own hairy-toothed mammoth. That kind of responsibility (say the experts) could easily put us off sex. So our orgasms are a kind of loyalty scheme, ensuring we come back for more and more and more. That theory is backed up by the clitoris itself, which serves no other purpose than to give us pleasure. In fact, it's the only organ in the human body whose function is purely to make us feel good. (Are you still convinced that God was a man? I'm not.)

Anyway, all this talk of orgasms isn't going to satisfy you at all if, despite determined, hands-on practice, you're not having any. Or if you're not having as many as you'd like. So let's recap with a quick lesson on how we have them, and how you can have more. It's a longer process than you'd imagine. Those 10 or so blissful seconds of pleasure you feel inside are actually the culmination of several stages.

Stage one: Arousal
During this stage your body starts preparing you to have sex, doing everything it can except putting on the Barry White CD, plumping up your duvet and lighting scented candles. Glands at the opening of your vagina (called Bartholin's glands, in case you would like to thank them personally) begin secreting lubricating juices, and blood rushes to your inner vaginal lips—making them darker in color and swollen. You might also notice a pink flush appear over your chest and neck. Your temperature rises, causing you to pant like a marathon runner, and your clitoris swells and hardens. Inside, you might feel achey and "empty"—this is because your vaginal walls have lengthened and opened in readiness for a penis. More glands inside you start producing even more lubricating fluid. This stage can take anything from 15 to 25 minutes to complete, by which time you'll be warm, pink, gasping for air and telling him that he's welcome to stay over.

Stage two: Plateau

An extension of the arousal phase, plateau sees you climbing the walls and begging him to "Get on with it." Your vagina keeps lengthening and opening up, and more lubrication is produced. Your clitoris becomes fully erect and super-sensitive to the touch. During sex, friction can pull the clitoral hood back (like a foreskin) and expose the inner bud. This is often almost unbearably sensitive to direct stimulation, but feels good when touched on the sides. The uterus shifts slightly backward, giving you more space in your vagina, and your cervix prepares for the onslaught of millions of spermazoids. Imagine parents waiting patiently outside a school for an outpouring of rowdy children, and you'll get the picture.

Stage three: Orgasm

Blood rushes to the chest, making nipples harden and breasts get bigger. Hurrah! The muscles inside the vaginal walls contract every 0.8 seconds (the same frequency as the ejaculations of a man's orgasm). The upper part of the vagina balloons out—to meet those pesky lil' sperms —and your breathing rate increases even more. By this point, you could need gas and air and a trained nurse on standby. After the first three to six seconds of contractions, the sensations begin to fade away, although the tissues remain engorged with blood—meaning that, with more stimulation, you can continue to orgasm.

Stage four: Resolution

Aaaah … and relax. Once the muscular contractions have stopped, the blood starts to drain away from your pelvic area. The vaginal lips and clitoris gradually begin to return to their prearousal size and color, and lubrication ceases altogether. Your heartbeat goes back to its normal rate, and your blood pressure begins to drop, which gives you a feeling of deep relaxation and often a fairly rapid need for sleep. You might well retain a slight pinky flush on your chest and face, and your mouth is probably swollen rather attractively. You suddenly notice that the man next to you in your bed is smiling at you proudly, and the neighbors are banging on the walls.

Different types of orgasm

More proof that women are superior to men at least in the orgasmic stakes is the fact that we can have different types of orgasm. Men only have two kinds—the normal kind, through stimulation of the penis, and the G-spot type when their prostate gland is directly stimulated. (We'll discuss those later). Poor things.

But with new erogenous zones being discovered every week, women have a whole smorgasbord of orgasms to choose from. It will probably soon be announced that we can orgasm from buying and breaking in a new pair of shoes. (And, if they're Manolos, it's true.) These may well be what you've experienced so far through direct clitoral stimulation. But it doesn't have to be stimulation by a hand or a tongue—you can achieve clitoral orgasms through sex. Here's how it happens.

The clitoris is much bigger than it looks. In fact, the visible bit is just the tip of the iceberg. It has nerve endings (crura) that extend along the labia majora and inside the vagina. During sex, these can be stimulated by the pressure of his penis, or his body moving against you.

Clitoral orgasms are described as: "Sharp, intense and about three seconds long." Psychoanalyst Sigmund Freud thought they were inferior to vaginal orgasms, for that reason. He found that women who experienced vaginal orgasms seemed more satisfied for longer. But what would he know? Did he ever have one?

Clitoral orgasms

How to have a clitoral orgasm: by yourself
This is covered in more detail in Chapter 1. Don't forget, fantasies are crucial, so conjure up the sexiest images you can. If bra-wearing spaniels dance through your brain, so be it. Don't edit your thoughts.

When your clitoris starts to become erect, standing away from the rest of your vagina and becoming hard, that's a sign that you're approaching orgasm, so keep going. Increase the pressure and pace until … until … oooh dear … bam!

Toys
You don't have to do all this hard work yourself. Actually, if you've never had an orgasm, I'd recommend you invest in a vibrator as soon as possible. They're marvelous. The following types are good for clitoral stimulation.

Standard vibrator: The small, handbag-sized basic models are ideal for beginners. They cost under $20 from sex shops and do the job nicely. Apply it to your clitoris, or to the sides of it, and feel those good vibrations sending you off to Orgasmville.

Massager: Your desert-island luxury has to be this type of handy, rechargeable pleasure-packer. More expensive than a normal vibrator (about $36), it comes with detachable heads so you can vary the sensations. They often have three speed settings : "Mmmm", "Oh God" and "My-panties-are-on-fire." You can also use it to massage your body and apply moisturizer to your face. But really, you won't want to.

Clitoral butterfly: I tried to make one of these once, by slipping an SOS pad into my pants. Did it work? Did it hell, so now I rely on the store-bought ones. They're a small, nobbly pad, shaped like a butterfly, that you slip down your panties onto your clitoris. You have a remote control to adjust the speed of the vibrations. Very, very nice and so discreet, you could wear it out shopping. A few people might notice you clinging to the walls and mouthing, "Oh sweet Jesus, help me," but you can just tell them you've noticed a really nice top on sale.

How to have a clitoral orgasm: with a friend
Try telling your lover that you've never had an orgasm before and you'd like him to help you have your first. That kind of challenge inspires some men; the others you can just pay. Lie down on the bed with your legs hanging over the edge of it. He can kneel on the floor in front of you, between your knees. This position works best as it almost feels as though you're alone, so you can concentrate purely on the sensations he is giving you. He should

start with gentle clitoral stimulation as described before. When your clitoris becomes hard, he can try the following technique.

Double-handed tongue teaser
He places both hands on your vagina, using the sides of his hands to pull apart your labia. As the clitoris is exposed, he presses a thumb on either side of it. He can then rub those thumbs up and down the sides of the clitoris (which is blissful), and then swirl his tongue over the clitoris itself (which is even better). Have him build up the pressure of his thumbs and tongue gradually, building up to him placing his mouth over the whole clitoris and licking it up and down. When you come, he can suck the clitoris into his mouth and shake his head from side to side, in a "No, no, no" motion—just as you start screaming, "Yes, yes, yes."

During sex
Perhaps the best position for a clitoral orgasm is woman on top. But not in the usual way. Instead of crouching over or straddling your man, lie directly on top of him. Brace your feet against his, keep your legs together and move yourself along his penis as you screw. This is so good because your clitoris comes into direct contact with his body—as you move back and forth, the clitoris is "sandwiched" between you and gets pulled and pushed with every thrust. By squeezing your legs together, you can get

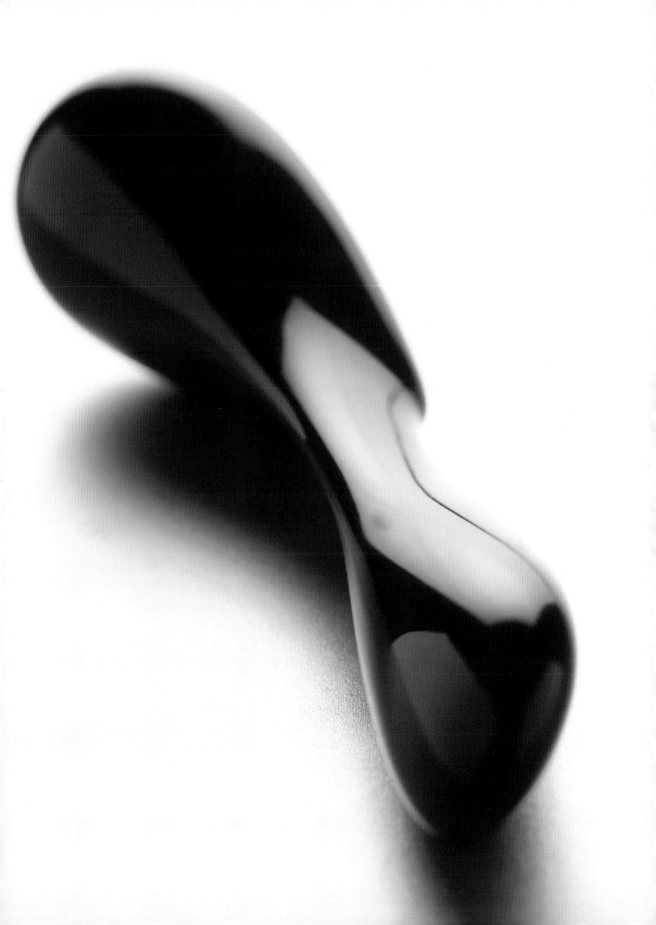

Love-eggs are sexy because they give your vagina that "filled up" feeling. They are also fabulous for exercising your PC muscles after you've had a baby.

The most boring-looking dildos can be the most satisfying. All you're looking for is width and length. Don't buy anything that would frighten your cleaning lady if she found it.

The best way to choose a sex toy is from other women's recommendations. Hold a sex toy party and encourage your friends to confess all. Or visit online sex shops—they often have anonymous reviews from pleased (or not so pleased) customers.

even more pressure going in your vulva, which should have the effect of stimulating you even further.

Missionary position: Another goodie is the missionary position, while you rub your clitoris with one hand—as long as his body is positioned so that your clitoris is within reach. This is successful for almost every woman who tries it. Don't be shy or panic that your partner will feel he's not enough. Men like women who take control of their pleasure. Honestly. (Besides, the majority of men find it darned sexy to watch a woman masturbate.)

Toys

Clit tickler: The name varies from store to store, but it's always the same deal: a knobbly ring that your man slides over his penis just prior to sex. The ring has soft nodules that rub against your clitoris while you screw. It works, it's cheap and your man will like it as it acts like a cock ring, keeping blood inside his penis for a stronger, longer erection.

Vibrating clit tickler: As you can guess, very similar to the abovementioned tickler, except with extra vibration. Probably more satisfying than the above but not as portable, as it has a remote control, connected to the ring by a long wire. Gets in the way a bit until you're used to

it. But do get used to it, as the vibrations feel very nice to both of you.

G-spot orgasms

The G-spot has caused controversy since it was first discovered by a German gynecologist Dr. Ernest Grafenberg and his (very happy) wife. Ever since then, scientists and couples have been searching for it avidly, with mixed results. Although many women would disagree, recent research claims it doesn't exist: in 2001, an American psychologist, Dr. Terence Hines, announced that Grafenberg's research had been limited and misleading. Grafenberg had, in fact, only tested 12 women for sensitivity in the area, and only 4 had said "Oooh!" I guess it depends on whether you choose to believe the claims of two male scientists or those of the many women who say they have actually experienced it.

Either way, it's got to be worth a try. Personally, I'm pretty convinced there is an area up there that feels darned good when it's rubbed the right way.

The G-spot is also often linked to female ejaculation, although it has been known for women to ejaculate from clitoral stimulation alone. According to the book *The G-Spot*, by Ladas, Whipple and Perry (Bantam Doubleday Dell, 1983), stimulation of the G-spot leads to ejaculation of fluid from the vagina. It's all very complicated and confusing. All I'll say is that anything that entices men to spend hours stimulating your vagina is a good thing and should be encouraged. Just put a towel down before you try.

Where is my G-spot?

Grafenberg claimed that the G-spot is situated about 2 inches inside the vagina, on the front wall. (That's the side of your vagina nearest your tummy.) It's an area of erectile tissue that some say feels flatter and smoother than the rest of the vaginal wall. It responds better to pressure than to actual rubbing.

How to have a G-spot orgasm:
by yourself

Toys

You could try to find your G-spot with your hands. If you use a diaphragm, sponge or cervical cap you are probably quite adept at manual exploration. Otherwise, you can invest in something that will make the search easier.

G-spot vibrator: Search any sex-toy catalog and you'll find hundreds of these—which at least suggests that there is an area up there that responds to stimulation. The best G-spot vibrators have a vibrating head on the end of a long, bendy neck. You just slip them in,

turn them on and—mmmm.

Your other choice is more dildo-like in appearance: the end of the vibrator is angled so that it hits the G-spot. Don't thrust it in and out, just hold it against the front wall of your vagina and let the vibrations do their thing. Otherwise angle a normal vibrator up towards your tummy, turn it on and have lots of fun.

Will I wet myself?

Only if you're doing it right. Most G-spot orgasms are preceded by the urge to pee. So that should be seen as a good sign—honestly—as it shows you're stimulating the right place (remember, it's found on the underside of the urethra). When you feel that urge, don't panic—just keep on stimulating the G-spot. This orgasm also differs from the clitoral one in that as you climax, you might feel like "pushing out" with your vaginal muscles. As you do, you may well notice that you release a lot of liquid. That's female ejaculation. Remember, it's not pee. So let go, honey, and ride those waves.

How to have a G-spot orgasm:
with a friend

Kneel on all fours and ask your lover (nicely) to insert two fingers inside you and then press down. If he notices a small area about 2 inches inside your vagina that feels different—more smooth, less ridged—than the rest, he's found your G-spot. Ask him to press down on it, moving his fingertips in very small, gentle circles. Don't let him push his fingers in and out of you like a reckless slot-machine player—tell him it's a small, pressing action. You should be in control here so you tell him what feels good. If nothing happens at all, get him to stimulate your clitoris at the same time. The G-spot should harden as you become more aroused, making it easier to find.

During sex

Any position as long as his penis reaches that front wall. Lots of couples have reported that doggy-style is a good one. Stay on all fours and have your partner repeat the above experiment with his penis. He should rotate his hips, grinding the head of his penis against your front vaginal wall. Don't let him go in too deep (as is a man's inclination)—remember, the G-spot is only about 2 inches inside you. When you start feeling the urge to come, push out with your vaginal muscles—he'll feel it against his penis and, with luck, you should climax together.

Toys

A little something that could well make G-spot sex even better for you is the studded condom. It has little nodules all along its length that can help stimulate your G-spot.

Multiple orgasms

To misquote that old country and western song, "Sometimes it's great to be a woman." When we have sex, for instance, because women have the ability to experience multiple orgasms and, if only for this reason, men will envy us forever. To explain why we have this wonderful capacity, we need to get a bit scientific, so tie your hair back and slap on some glasses and continue …

Why women can have multiple orgasms and men (usually) can't

It's all down to the refractory period. This is the period immediately following ejaculation where men always want a snooze. His penis is supersensitive and he physically cannot come. He usually loses his erection too. (There's probably a medical reason for this period, like his testes need a break to restock the semen supplies, but I don't know for sure.) The length of time it lasts depends on his age—younger men can have a very short refractory period (around 20 minutes), while older men might need a couple of days between getting laid. However, women don't have a refractory period. We don't need a break between orgasms—our bodies are capable of climaxing over and over again. Good news? You betcha! There's nothing to stop you having multiple orgasms tonight and every night following. Want some of that? Then here's how to do it.

We have the most fantastic sex toys attached to our bodies—o

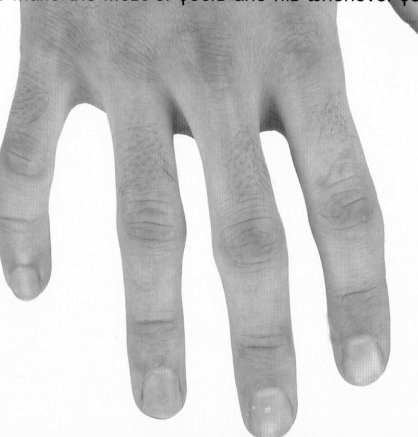

ands—so make the most of yours and his whenever you can.

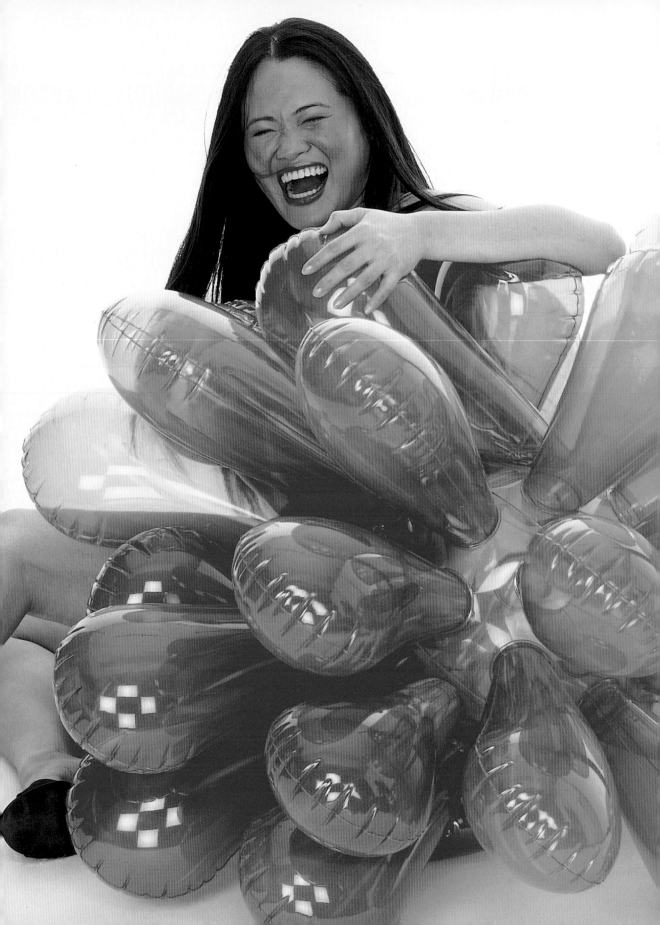

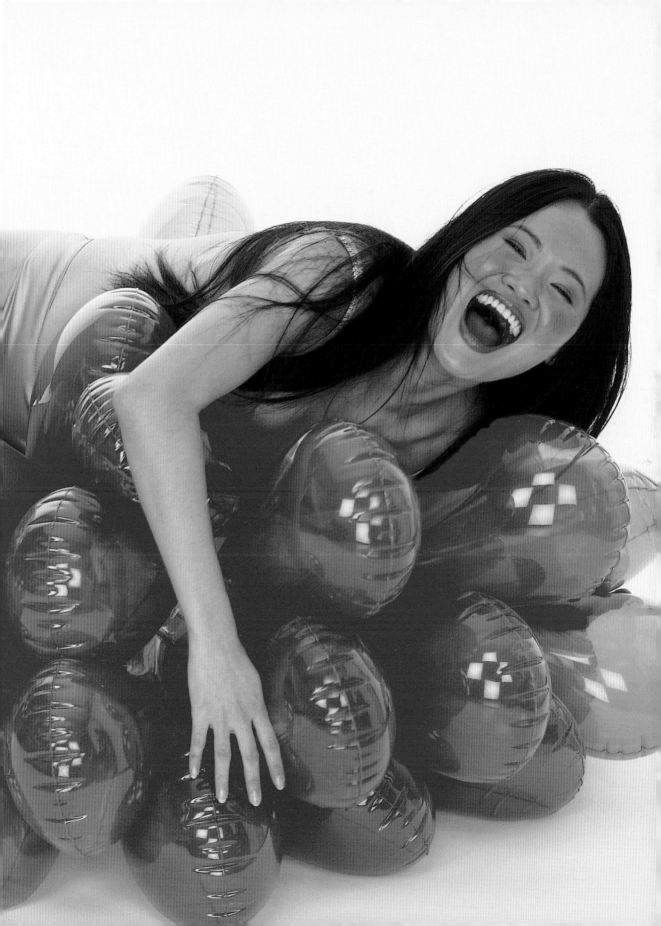

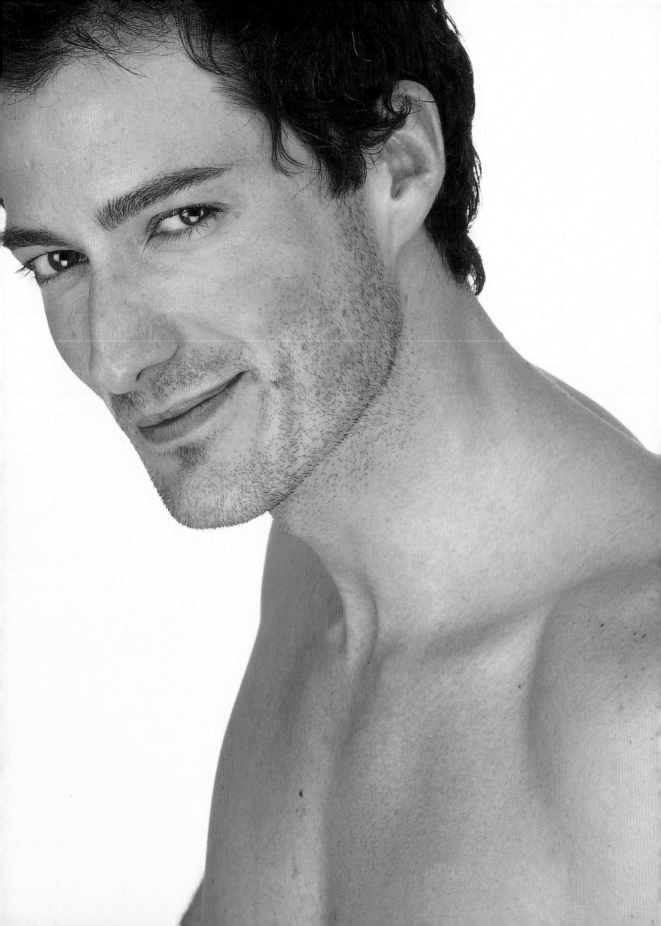

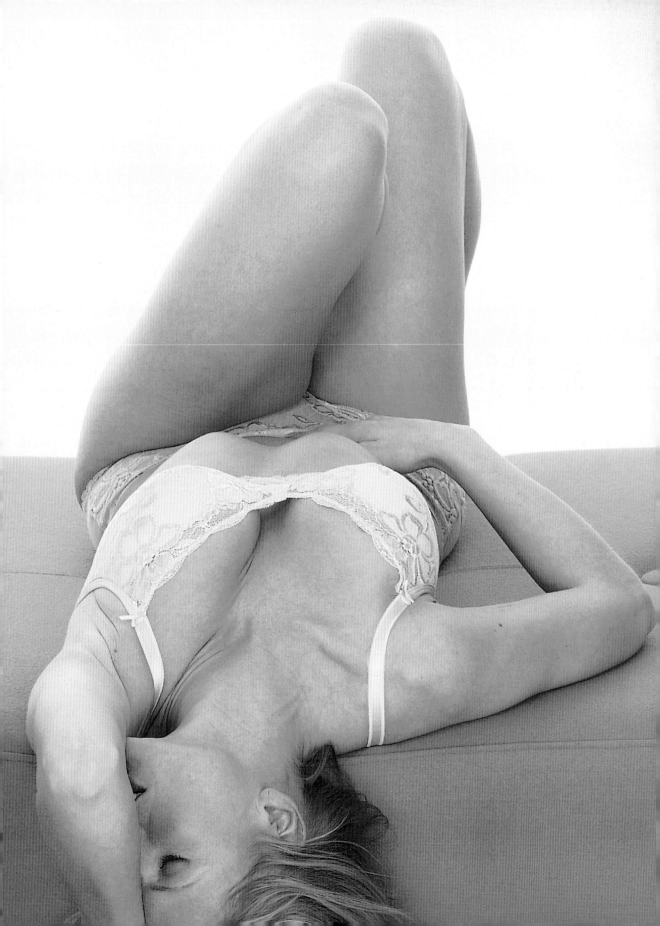

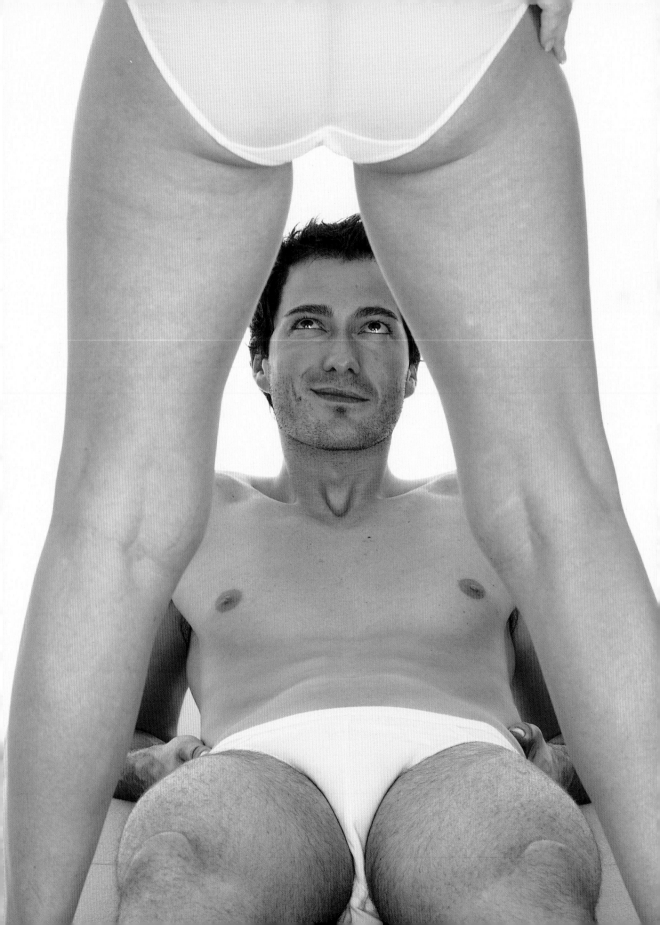

How to have a multiple orgasm:
by yourself

Start masturbating like a mad woman. Do everything you can to bring yourself to a climax. As your orgasm builds, go with it. Flail, thrash, claw the pillow—aaahh. Bliss. Then keep going. At first you'll probably hate it: your clitoris will feel overly sensitive, you won't be able to bear the sensation. But don't give up. Vary your technique a bit so you're not concentrating directly on the clitoris—try the sides, or underneath. But whatever you do, keep going and keep masturbating.

After a while, you'll start to feel the sensations coming again. Again, allow yourself to come. It might feel different from the first orgasm, either stronger or weaker. Most multiple orgasm devotees say the pattern is: first orgasm—strong, second orgasm—weak, third orgasm—very strong, fourth orgasm—awesome, fifth orgasm—quite strong. (Nobody said what happened after that. I suspect they never quite found the strength to aim for number six.)

How to have a multiple orgasm:
with a friend

Most men adore helping you multiple orgasm, although they can get jealous. (Don't worry, just offer to lend him your car afterwards.)

Start by enjoying lots of foreplay. You should aim to have your first orgasm before you have sex, so have him go down on you or use a vibrator to stimulate your clitoris. Then start having sex, and masturbate yourself as you do, until you have the second orgasm. Change positions, to vary the sensation, and just keep going. There's no big secret—you just have to keep experiencing strong, varied stimulation. After he's come, he can masturbate you to the final climax.

What stops orgasms?

Even if you're getting exactly the right kind of stimulation, sometimes you just can't orgasm. It's a drag but it's normal. Women are more prone to this than men because we tend to carry our emotional life around with us all the time, and the cause of this is usually an emotional problem of some sort.

There are some pills and medicines that can inhibit orgasms. But it's perfectly normal to have a few sessions without being able to come, even if you're totally healthy.

The key is if you are worried, take the pressure off altogether. Either concentrate on giving him great oral sex—he won't mind a bit—or try taking a break from sex. In the meantime continue to boost your sensuality (see Chapter 1) and your partner's.

Q+A

■ **I want to orgasm at the same time as my partner during sex. Is there an easy way?**

■ **The orgasms I have with my partner are never as intense as the ones I have alone. It's not his fault —he does everything right. So what's my problem?**

● Aaah—the elusive simultaneous orgasm. So common in films, so rare in reality. If you went to see a sexual therapist about this, they'd tell you it's probably not worth aiming for. But what do they know? Okay, the secret is loads of foreplay. Basically, you (the woman) need to be as near to orgasm as possible before you start screwing. So do anything it takes to get really aroused. I mean, really, duvet-clawingly, knuckle-chewingly aroused. Then, when you start having sex, concentrate on how good it feels. Tell him how good it feels. Tell him how close you are to coming. When you're really close, tell him, and tell him he has permission to come. Then let yourself go. You should both get there at the same time. If that seems complicated, or you're embarrassed to talk to him during sex, just remember the basic idea is to time your orgasm to coincide with his. If he normally comes quickly, make sure you're right on the edge before you start. If he lasts quite a while, you needn't be so worked up.

● You're probably feeling inhibited when you climax in front of him. Let's face it, when you're flailing away on your own, you can totally let yourself go. You can also pace yourself so you build slowly and steadily towards your orgasm. With a guy, you could be feeling pressured to come, that he might be getting impatient, or you might simply be feeling like you're on show. There are cures however. The first is to draw the curtains. Sex in the dark is much more exciting for some women because their partner can't see their reactions. (Men dislike it for exactly that reason.) Try doing it in blackness and see if it allows you to concentrate better on coming. Next, encourage your man to build more slowly towards your orgasm. Be sure he gives you plenty of foreplay, hours of it, so you're really and truly aroused. And last, just relax a bit. You'll never know how erotic men find it to watch a woman orgasm. Let yourself go a little more.

You wouldn't believe how erotic men find it to watch a woman

■ I never come. Ever. Am I a freak?

● No. Don't worry—they're not going to cart you away to the circus. Sadly, many women find it incredibly difficult to orgasm. In my oh-so-wide experience, I've found it usually comes down to three things. First, lack of clitoral stimulation. Have you ever masturbated with a vibrator? It's the quickest way to orgasm for many women as it delivers precision stimulation to exactly the right spot. The clitoris barely gets any attention during normal sex, which might explain why you never "get there." Buy a cheap vibrator (one of the handbag-sized models we discussed earlier), and lock yourself in your bedroom for a weekend. Still nothing? Then you might have emotional worries. Ask yourself—do you feel guilty? Do you feel unattractive or unworthy of an orgasm? Do you feel "naughty," or that you shouldn't come? If you do, then please see a counselor. If you don't have any of these worries but you still don't come, you might have a fetish. Again, try masturbating with a vibrator but let your thoughts run wild. Think of anything and everything—from bondage to exhibitionism. You might spot a trigger.

■ My friends say that they have really strong contractions during orgasms. I don't. What's up with that?

● You might just have slightly weaker PC muscles than your friends. Some (very lucky) women do have superstrong contractions during orgasms, some have mild ones and some, like you, can barely feel theirs. Everyone is normal. Try doing your Kegel exercises more regularly (p. 146) and you might feel a difference.

rgasm. Let yourself go a little more.

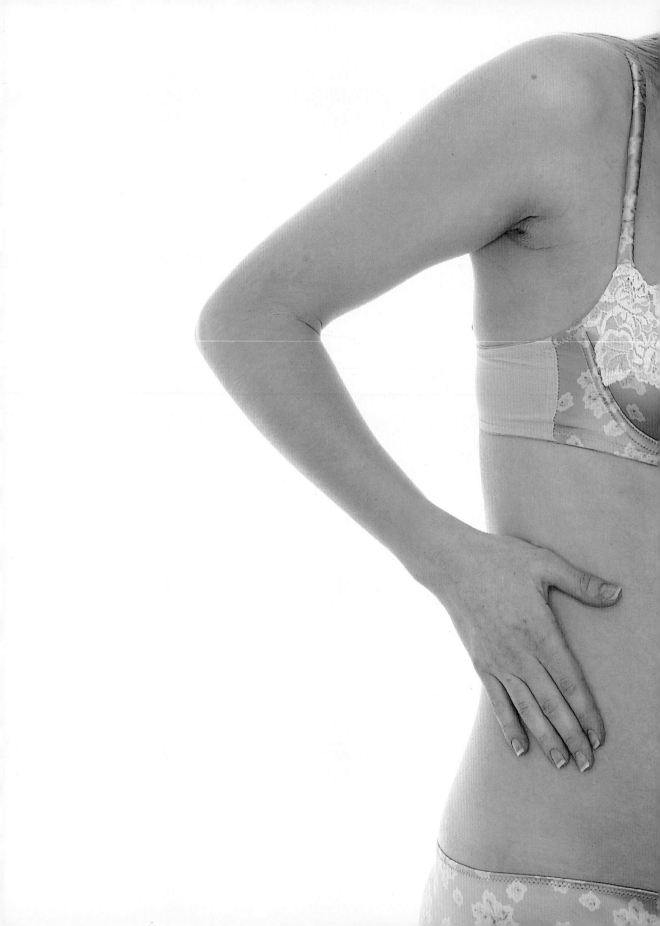

7 You sexy mother

(where babies come from)

Personal story: Sex for a baby is the sexiest sex!

I never particularly wanted to have children. I was a career girl. But when I met Simon, all that changed. I'd find myself smiling as I walked past parks with swings, and I'd give harassed mothers a hand carrying their strollers up the subway escalators.

Simon wanted children. It was one of the things I liked about him — I got quite misty-eyed when he said that his dream was to have a huge old farmhouse with loads of kids running around. A year later we were married and the conversations started to get more specific. We both decided we'd start trying for a baby after a year.

At around the same time, a friend of mine had just had a baby. She said it was fun. I was surprised. People usually sigh wearily and mumble that it's "hard work, but worth it." I told Simon that I thought we should start trying, arguing that, as we were both hopelessly unhealthy, it would take us years to conceive. We ended that conversation in bed.

It was so sexy trying for a baby. That's another thing nobody tells you — sex for a baby is the sexiest sex! I felt laid open, exposed, like I was this Earth Mother receptacle waiting to be filled up with Simon's sperm. Luckily I didn't tell him that, or we'd probably never have done it again.

We were lucky. I got pregnant immediately. For about two weeks afterwards we were still screwing unstoppably. It was partly elation at how fertile we were — Simon felt like a "caveman," he said. Nine months later, Jack was born.

Anne, 33

Where babies come from

Do you know? Don't be ashamed or embarrassed if you don't. I wasn't 100 percent sure until I started researching this chapter. The only time we get told is when we're 15 at school, and most of that knowledge gets buried under the more pressing issues of hairspray and eyeliner. The age that we really need reproduction lessons is 25—the average age when women in the United States have their first child.

So here are the facts. When a man and a woman love each other very much—or, at least, when a man and a woman finally realize that they're stuck with each other, have nothing to talk about any more and can't think of anything else to give each other for Christmas—they have sex. Millions of sperm are released from the man's penis (usually accompanied by shouts of, "I'm coming, baby!") into the woman's vagina. Here they travel up, pass through the small opening to the uterus at the top—the cervix—and finally reach her fallopian tubes.

Here, all the sperm hang around for a bit, nudging each other competitively. If the couple has got their timing right, an egg has just been released from one of her ovaries and floats down into one fallopian tube where all the little guys are waiting, like teenagers outside a 7-Eleven.

The sperm surge forward and attack the egg. Enzymes inside the sperm's head eat away at the egg's lining, and one of them manages to break through. Once a sperm has made it inside the egg, the egg is "fertilized." No other sperm can get into the egg now. Then the fertilized egg floats down to the uterus, where it embeds itself into the wall and starts to grow.

That's the theory anyway. In truth, a lot can go wrong at every stage of the process, which is why the scientists say there is only a 25 percent chance of successful conception in any given month. The sperm can fail to make it through the cervix (in fact, only 0.1 percent actually ever do). Or they can make it through, but then die before the egg makes it to the rendezvous point. Even if sperm and egg meet, the egg might not be fertilized. And even if it is, it can fail to embed itself in the uterus and just be expelled with the next period. Sometimes the body goes on to realize that there's a fault somewhere, and terminates ("miscarries") the pregnancy.

The waiting game

When you're 15, you are given the impression that you can get pregnant if you so much as sit next to a boy on the bus. But the truth is, you almost can at that age. We're ridiculously fertile in our teens, and get progressively less so as we get older. Sadly, our chances of conceiving fall to just 10 percent by the time we're 35. Which is usually the age when we've sorted out our lives enough to finally want loads of plastic stuff strewn around our living rooms.

The reason we get less fertile is our eggs. They have a sell-by date stamped on them, and it says "Best before 35." We are born with all our eggs already in our ovaries—about two million—and they go off a bit every year. This is why career women choose to get some eggs frozen when they're still young. Men's sperm, however, are created fresh every day until they die, which is why they can still father children even when their dicks are covered in liver-spots and surrounded by white pubic hairs. Life is completely unfair.

The fertility cycle

If you want to get pregnant, the first thing to do is buy yourself a diary. Well, no—the first thing to do is meet a man, wait for him to call, go on a few dates, get to know him as a person, make a commitment to each other, work through a couple of arguments, go on holiday and buy a house with a spare bedroom. *Then* buy a diary. You'll need to know your fertility cycle, which means tracking your periods.

Every woman is different, but the average menstrual cycle lasts around 28 days and ovulation (when the egg is released, ready to be fertilized) is roughly in the middle, about 14 days before the next period. A woman often gets pregnant through intercourse just before ovulation, because sperm can live happily inside her for up to 48 hours, effectively "waiting" there to fertilize her egg.

Wait for your next period and when it arrives—usually when you're miles from your bathroom and wearing white pants—mark it in your diary. This is Day 1 of your cycle. From Days 11 to 15, screw like you've never screwed before. Then—repeat.

Some women (like my friend Anita) can actually feel when they ovulate—she says it's a dull, grindy ache low down in her abdomen. I can't. But there are other ways to tell when you're fertile. As well as tracking your periods, you can examine your vaginal mucus.

Examining your vaginal mucus

Trust me, when you're actually giving birth you'll have to do much worse things, so you might as well get used to it now. What happens is this: vaginal discharge is usually pretty scarce, and of a sticky consistency, but when you ovulate it changes to a thin, stringy consistency. This is to help those brave little spermazoids travel up your vagina. Wait till you hit day 11 of your cycle, then look at your panties or push two fingers inside you, first thing in the morning, and examine what you get. If you are producing thin, stringy juices that stretch between your fingers like egg whites, you are ovulating. Go forth and get laid, young woman. But if it's still thick and more "glue-y," save your strength and try again tomorrow. If it's yellow and smelly, you might have a yeast infection.

Sex to get pregnant

Another method is to take your temperature. Using a basal body thermometer first thing in the morning (ask your doctor), you can measure the changes in temperature that occur when you ovulate. It rises by 0.2–0.6 degrees when you're ready to conceive, and either stays at that level if you get pregnant, or falls again after ovulation if you don't. Products are in development that track your temperature using a thermometer you wear on your wrist like a watch. (Not something to wear on a first date.)

Another, less scientific but much more fun, way to predict your ovulation date is to watch who you are attracted to. Most of the time we are attracted to men who would make good fathers. This means steady men, reliable ones, who aren't likely to forget where we live or to bring home food. But when we are ovulating—forget it. Our penchant for Mr. Nice goes out the window and we are attracted, for those three or four crucial baby-making days, to quite another type of man. The fertile man. In normal speech, big hunks. Great big tall, strong, rugged men with symmetrical features (symmetrical equals fertile in the dating world) who could knock us up as quick as look at us. While you're tracking your periods in your diary, look out for who you lech after. When you notice that you're suddenly spending an inordinate amount of time hanging round building sites, or that you're shouting suggestive remarks back at them, get under a duvet and start screwing immediately.

But how do you screw when you want to make a baby? I've known some women who were very soppy about the whole thing. My friend Sarah was the worst: "We wanted the whole thing to be romantic, so we lit candles and told each other how much we loved each other before we began. Then we tried to make the night very special and intimate, with lots of handholding and kisses. Finally, we lay in bed afterwards and talked about what our baby might be like."

Get me a bucket. Of course, none of that nonsense worked. What finally did the trick was Sarah's husband coming home drunk from a Christmas party and leaping on her while she was bent over scrubbing the kitchen floor. Romantic? No. Primal, animal-style fucking? Yes. And that's what you want to achieve to make yourself a baby. If, for any reason, you plan on telling your child about its conception, you can always fib and say it was a very special lovely moment. But Mother Nature isn't too bothered about candles and whispered compliments. She just wants that sperm pumped as far up your insides as possible.

So, here, in reverse order, is the Best Position For Baby-Making Top Three:

Spoons
In this position, the couple is their most relaxed and so more easily achieve orgasm. It's also quite good for achieving the depth that a man needs to really fire those baby-bullets up there.

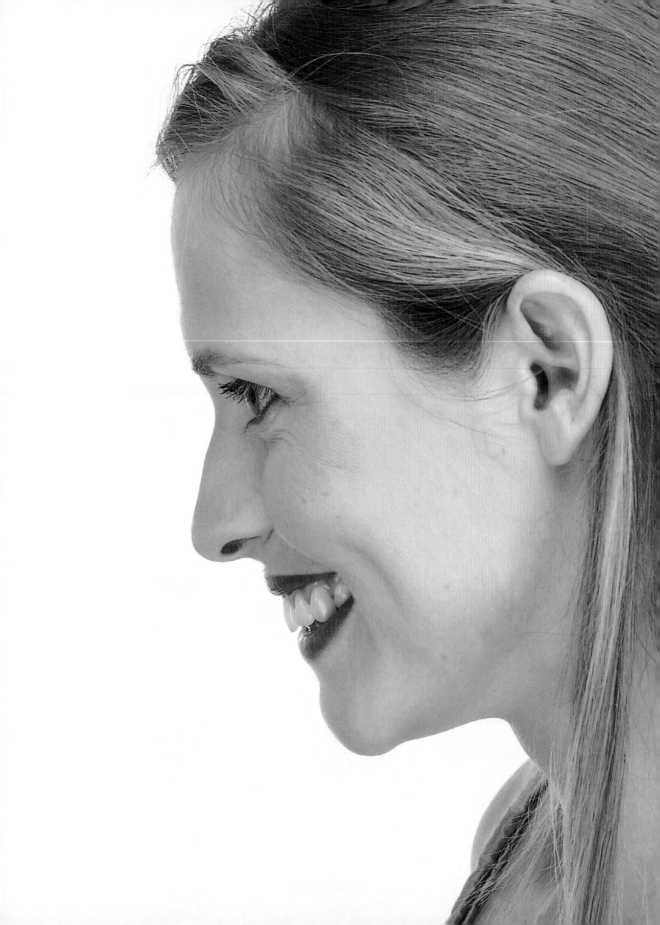

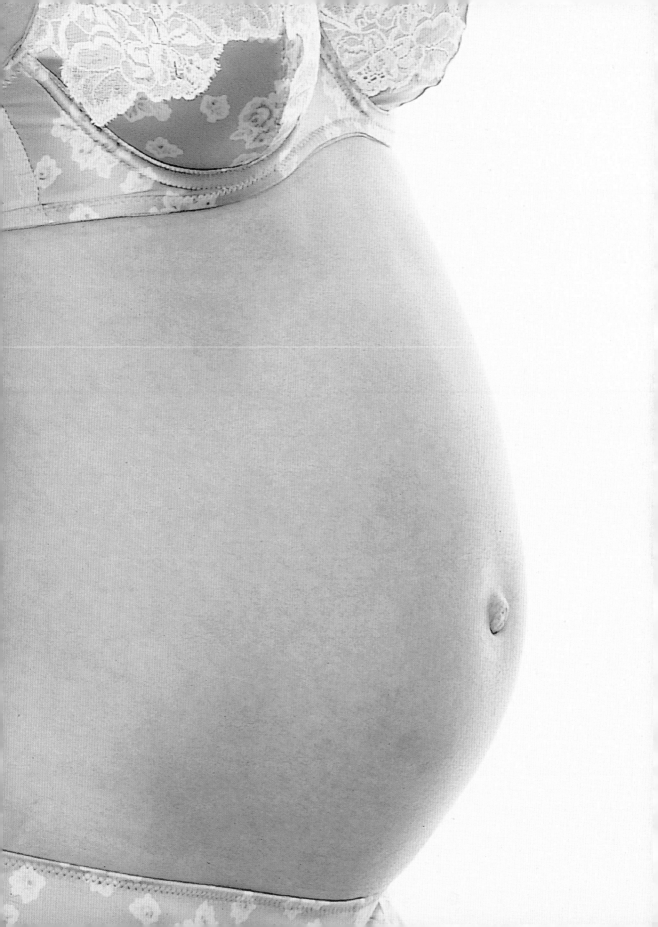

Doggy

About as non-face-strokey as you can get. But brilliant for baby-making as the man gets depth. You know how sometimes it can actually hurt slightly, as his dick can bang against the top of your vagina? That's what you want, darling, so bite that pillow and tell yourself it's nothing compared to childbirth. (Am I helping?)

Missionary position

Okay, this is quite romantic. At least you can gaze into each other's eyes. But that's not why it works. It works because, if you raise your legs during the sex, your vagina is shortened and the sperm have a shorter distance to travel. Also, you (the woman) are more likely to orgasm in this position, and that helps a lot. With each contraction of your vaginal walls, the sperm get pushed up toward your cervix. Like little surfers. Bless 'em. Pillows under your butt also help, tilting your vagina up.

The worst positions? That's easy. Don't go on top—his sperm will just trickle out of you and ruin your chances of motherhood, and your sheets. Don't try anything really acrobatic like standing up, for the same reason. Obviously, anal isn't the way to go.

But I want a boy!

Oh, God. This is where we step off the path and wander into old wives territory. There are many superstitions about how you affect the sex of your child. Some are based on scientific fact, especially those about foods to eat or when to have sex. The pH level of your vagina matters, which depends on diet, whether you are on antibiotics and where you are in your life cycle—boy sperm prefer a more alkaline pH level in your vagina, so eating red meat and salty foods can encourage little-boy sperm on their quest. Girls prefer a degree of acidity, although not too much—this kills off sperm altogether.

Also, boy sperms aren't as strong as girl sperms. Boys can swim faster, but they die if left to hang around too long with no egg to fertilize. (Just picture men waiting in stores and you'll get the idea.) So, for a boy, screw on the day you ovulate or up to 24 hours afterwards. That'll give them a chance to zoom up your insides and hit the egg while it's waiting there. For a girl, screw earlier, up to three days before you ovulate. Girl sperms are happy to wait around and they'll meet the egg when it finally appears.

These are the only even vaguely rational tips. The rest—which I'll list anyway—are sheer nonsense, but just prove what we'll believe when our hormones are humming.

Sex during pregnancy

For a boy

● Focus on his pleasure—if the male climaxes first, you're supposedly guaranteed a son.

● Give in to seduction—if the man is the one to suggest some baby-making, you'll get a boy.

● Sleep to the left of your partner.

● Make love when a quarter moon is in the sky.

● Have sex at night.

● Mark your calendar—more boys are conceived on odd days of the month.

● Follow the compass—pointing the woman's head north while you make love "guarantees a boy" says an insane friend of mine (with, okay, three sons).

For a girl

● Focus on her pleasure—if the woman orgasms before her partner, you can decorate your nursery in pink.

● Take the lead—if the woman initiates sex, you'll get a girl.

● Make a date for love in the afternoon.

● Get together on the even days of the month.

So there you are, you old wife. You've made love on the 17th of the month, it was a full moon and your head banged against the headboard in the southwestern corner of the room … Or something. Anyway, you're pregnant. Is this the end of your sex life as you know it?

In a word—maybe.

It depends. All I can give you is my own experience on this one. For the first three months I wasn't particularly interested in sex for the simple reason that my head was usually halfway down a lavatory and I've never found the words "American Standard" particularly erotic. My man wasn't too enthralled either—he was terrified of killing the baby—so we didn't get up to much. But in the fourth month—woohoo! Nobody tells you this, but when you're pregnant, you get vastly increased blood-flow to your vagina. It's all getting pumped down there to help with all the baby growing that's going on. You can actually feel the change, as your private parts are "fuller" and you get a lot more lubricated.

Is that good? You betcha! With all that blood racing around, my potential for orgasms tripled overnight. The clitoris is much, much more sensitive when you're pregnant and I could hit the spot just from crossing my legs. Also, my boobs supersized themselves, and my stomach was still relatively flat. All in all, I don't think we left the bedroom except to get the papers and a bottle or two of Gatorade.

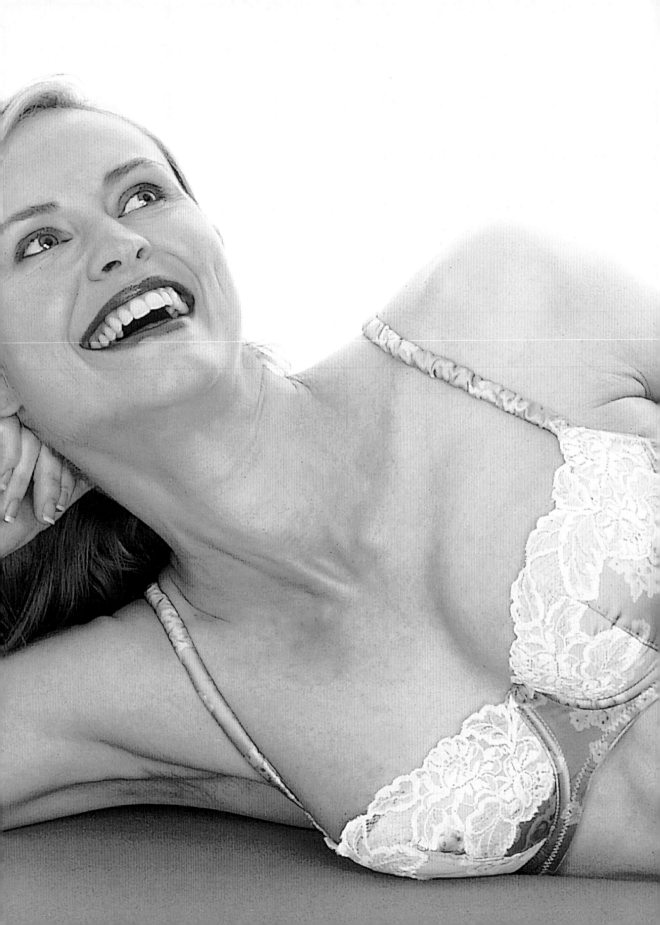

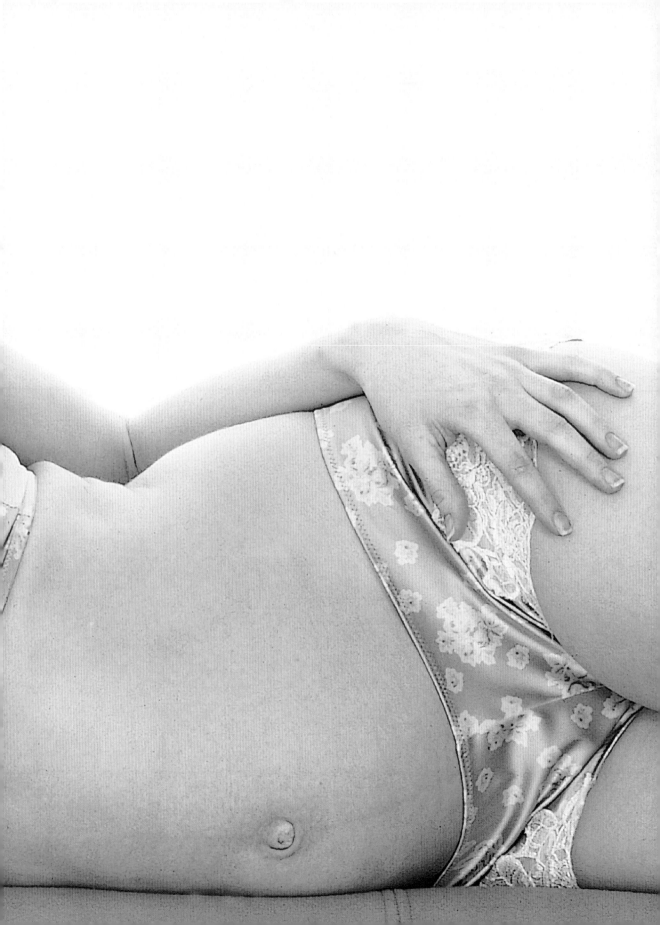

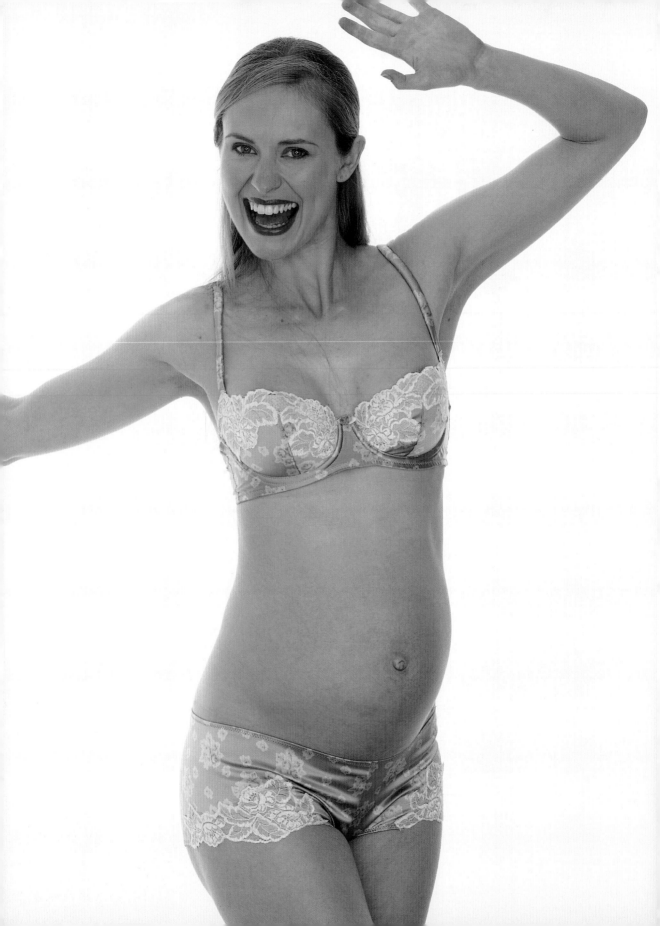

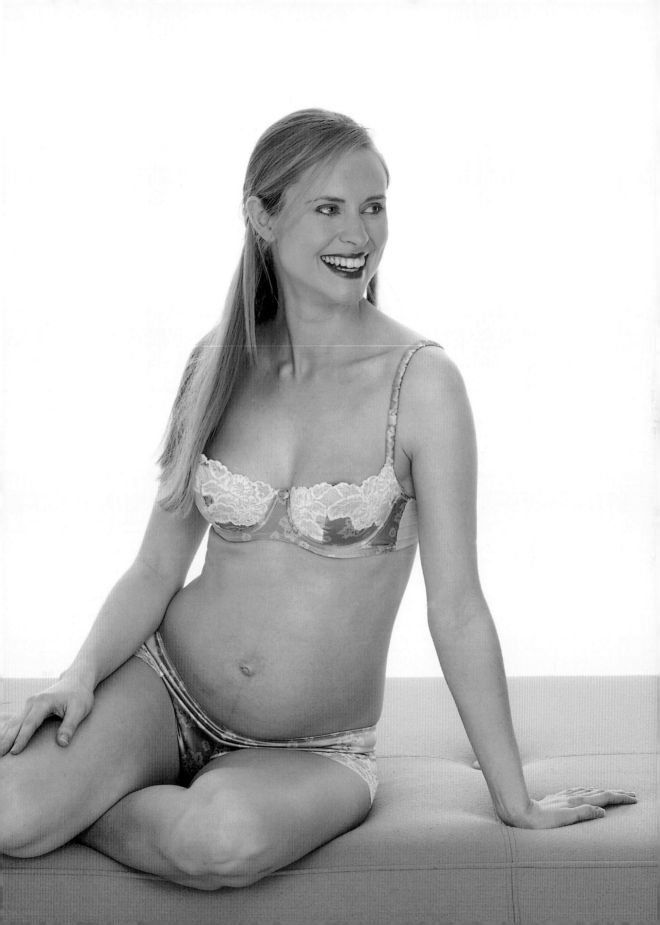

Sex after pregnancy

In the fifth and sixth months, my stomach started ballooning and it was becoming very apparent that I was pregnant. Of course, we knew I was pregnant, but you can still make yourselves forget, on purpose, so as not to put yourselves off. It was around this time that we dropped the man-on-top positions.

And in the final trimester (the last three months), it dwindled. This was my man's fault. He felt like he was being watched from inside me and completely lost the urge. I, on the other hand, could still blank out the baby during sex—even though my stomach was now of mammoth proportions. To be frank, I would have done it right up until the birth itself. I'm not a pervert, but the blood-flow thang was sooooo strong and the hormones raging so hard that sex was amazing.

Whether you have sex or don't during your pregnancy depends on the pair of you and how your pregnancy is going. For example, if you've had any blood loss during the first weeks, or if you have a history of miscarriage, you'll be advised by your doctor to lay off the love-ins until the "danger time" (the first 12 weeks) has passed. However, at the very end of your pregnancy, your doctor might encourage you to screw like rabbits to bring on the birth. Sperm contains the same hormone, prostaglandin, that they use to induce labor. There's nothing like a good session to get that baby in gear.

When you're pregnant, there's so much going on that your hands are full whether you screw or not. The big change happens afterwards.

One of the worst jobs in the world must be Contraception Adviser on a maternity ward. Some have them, it's usually a young doctor, and they go from bed to bed asking new mothers what method of contraception they'll be using in the future. It's a valid exercise, but terrifying. All you can hear are jeers, screams, and shouts of, "If you think that I'm ever letting a penis near me again …" which are rapidly ended with a water jug being flung at the poor guy.

You're not allowed to have sex for six weeks after you've dropped. Which, believe me, is fine. For one thing, you hurt. (Or you're terrified of popping your stitches.) And for another, you are laid low with a monster period that starts on the Happy Day and carries on gushing for a week or so. It's all the womb lining and placenta and … you don't want to know. Just buy some disposable pants for your baby bag and wait and see.

Then you have your six-week checkup with the doctor. She examines your baby, then she examines you. She asks how you're sleeping, you laugh hollowly, and then she ends the appointment with the cheerful announcement: "You can now have sex again."

My doctor was funny. She followed it up with, "… but you might want to wait until you get home." But still, I wasn't laughing. I knew it would be a long time before I got horny again. Apart from the physical changes, my mental attitude towards sex had changed for the moment. I felt hideous. My boobs were full of milk, and my stomach was still looking about five months pregnant. I'd had a cesarean, so my privates weren't damaged.

My husband too, was fazed. We had a baby, I was a mother, youth had ended and respon-sibilities had crowded in. When he looked at me, he didn't see a sexual partner. He saw a tired, stressed-out zombie in a robe covered in baby barf. It took three months (and burning that robe) to get back on track.

But we did. And that's the message here: you will have sex again. And it'll be just as good as before. Just heed the following advice:

You sexy mother—hints and tips

1. Lose the extra weight

I know, I sound like the Fashion Mafia, but the truth is you won't feel sexy until you feel you look sexy. For me, that wasn't until I'd joined a diet club and lost 20 pounds. When your clothes start fitting again, that's when you'll feel sexy. You might be lucky and lose all the weight in a week. But if you don't, start cutting out sugary snacks and lock up the cookies. It's worth it. Even try and do a bit of exercise. You can go for long walks with your baby.

2. Give yourself the first three months off

Scientists believe that a human baby actually requires 12 months' gestation before it's fully formed. It's only born at nine months because your pelvis is physically too small to allow anything bigger to pass through. And when you have a baby, you'll still feel pregnant until it's three months old. Those first 12 weeks are draining—the baby needs you, and your milk, day and night. Can you fit in sex?

3. Be nice to each other

It's so easy to be irritable and so hard not to be. You're tired; he's tired. The only one of you who ever gets any sleep is the baby, and all three of you are madly disoriented. My midwife told me, with scary formality, that "marital harmony is severely reduced after the birth of a child" and warned that unless I stopped snapping at my husband like a rabid terrier, he might leave. She was right, of course. And luckily she was so strict that I listened and we all managed to get through it. Yes, obviously your partner won't do stuff for the baby either as well or efficiently as you do. That's Nature. But if you want a happy partnership, don't tell him that, and let him get on with doing things his way. This is a difficult time for fathers as there is little for them to do.

4. Don't expect mad sex until the baby sleeps in his or her own room

It didn't put me off to have my son lying there next to us in his Moses basket, but it wasn't the sexiest location in the world. However, the risk of crib death is reduced by a huge amount if the baby sleeps in your room for its first six months. I think it's worth having the baby in the bedroom for that long, and just making the living room the place where all the magic happens.

5. Don't gripe about your partner to your child when the baby monitor is switched on

Something I wish I'd known.

6. Be aware of postnatal depression

Weird though it sounds, if you get PND, you might be the last person to realize. It's like PMS—all the signs are there, but you don't actually make the mental leap into realizing that there's something wrong and you are feeling awful. PND is different from the "baby blues." Baby blues usually kick in around the third or fourth day after the birth, when your estrogen and progesterone levels suddenly dip. Almost all women suffer (and so, almost all men do too)—the symptoms are weepiness, anticlimax, exhaustion and a tendency to throw bunches of flowers at well-meaning visitors. Don't even try to fight it. Just use it (like I did) to get moved to your own room in the hospital.

Postnatal depression is much harder to cope with. Your doctor will look out for the signs, so don't think you have to monitor it all by yourself. It usually starts a couple of weeks after the birth, and the symptoms can be frightening. Extreme tiredness, mixed with a feeling of hopelessness and helplessness. Anger towards the baby, or severe overprotectiveness. Anxiety—worries that the baby is desperately ill when he seems fine to everyone else. Feeling that you can't get out of bed, and that you wish the baby would just go away. And, most of all, a terror that nobody could possibly understand.

They can understand. Postnatal depression is a real, medical disorder that affects the lives of some mothers. Please believe that you can tell someone about it: your partner, your doctor, a friend or a health visitor. It's medical. You're not a bad mother if you get it. Some women believe most mothers suffer a form of post-traumatic stress after giving birth, and that antidepressants can help greatly. Just do whatever you can to get help. (It's worth noting that if you have a history of depression, you're slightly more likely to get PND. But really, it can happen to anyone.) There are associations that will help you; consult your doctor, call a local helpline.

7. Accept that you are obsessed with your baby and will be for some time

So what if, when your partner starts lovingly licking your elbow, all you can think about is when Junior's next feed is due? That's normal. I mean, don't go mad—don't actually *tell* your partner that's what's on your mind. But don't beat yourself up over it either. You are programed to be completely immersed in your baby. You will be forever, but right now it's new and more than a little alarming. (When you're 70, your partner will be licking your elbow and you'll be wondering how Junior is coping with your grandkids ... or perhaps why it is that your partner still doesn't know your hotspots after 50 years of marriage.)

We all know that some mothers are obsessed with their kids to an annoying level. When you try to make conversation with them, their eyes wander towards their sleeping infant and, if it dares even fart in its sleep, she'll be panicking about gastroenteritis. Yes, they're annoying. But don't feel you have to swing the other way and be a hip young mom who can still talk Jimmy Choo shoes while their baby screams in the background. There is a happy medium. If need be, surround yourself with fellow moms for the first few months and make contact with your single girlfriends later.

8. Get a babysitter

You'll read, in the mountain of literature that you receive when you've had a baby, that making time for just you and your partner is a good idea. You'll read it, and you'll ignore it. No new mother can ever put their partner before their child. Relax—you don't have to.

I'm certainly not going to make you. But I will suggest that you pretend a bit.

After about four months, your partner will start trying to get you back into the real world. He might suggest that you leave the baby with your mom for a weekend. He might suggest that you start wearing real clothes again. Whatever he does, agree. It's the father's job to drag the new mother back into the land of the living.

And when he eventually succeeds in his mission, and you find yourself there—blinking in the restaurant like a young fawn—you'll actually be quite pleased about it. You never know, you might even want to have sex when you get home. No pressure. But you might.

9. Get a babyless friend to take you clothes shopping

Something strange happens when you're pregnant—you stop caring about clothes. Nothing fits you anyway, nice maternity clothes cost a fortune, and the ones you can buy fairly cheaply actually induce morning sickness in everyone who sees you wearing them.

Most women live in their partner's shirts and track pants for the duration. But about four months after the birth, when clothes start to fit again, you'll realize that fashion has been marching on and you have no idea what to wear. Nothing makes you feel worse. You! Who always knew the right shoe to wear. You! Who bought a handkerchief top three months before Posh

Spice did. Suddenly you have no idea if it's flat shoes or stilettos, and if eyeliner is now heavy or non-existent. What to do?

Go shopping, without the baby, with a friend who hasn't just created a human life. When you come back home loaded with shopping bags and try on your new outfits in front of your new family (lying, obviously, about their cost), everyone will feel you're back to normal. Including you.

If you can't afford new clothes, beg, steal or borrow them from friends. Tell people who are dying to give gifts that your baby has loads—it's you who needs a new top. Cry to your mom if necessary. Just do it. Because when you feel you look sexy, you know what happens: you are.

Protect yourself

In the craziest bit of Mother Nature's logic ever (who says she's a woman?), your fertility can be at its all-time peak after you give birth. For the next three months, your body is just desperate to make more babies. This is crazy, as it's actually not good for you to have babies back-to-back. So, remember your contraception. When they come round to talk about it in the hospital, try not to throw things and do try to listen. New options are available now—IUDs are good for women who've had babies, while, if you've previously used a diaphragm, you'll need to get it refitted. Don't rely on "just not doing it." You never know, one day you might want to. (Don't shout at me! I'm only saying you might!)

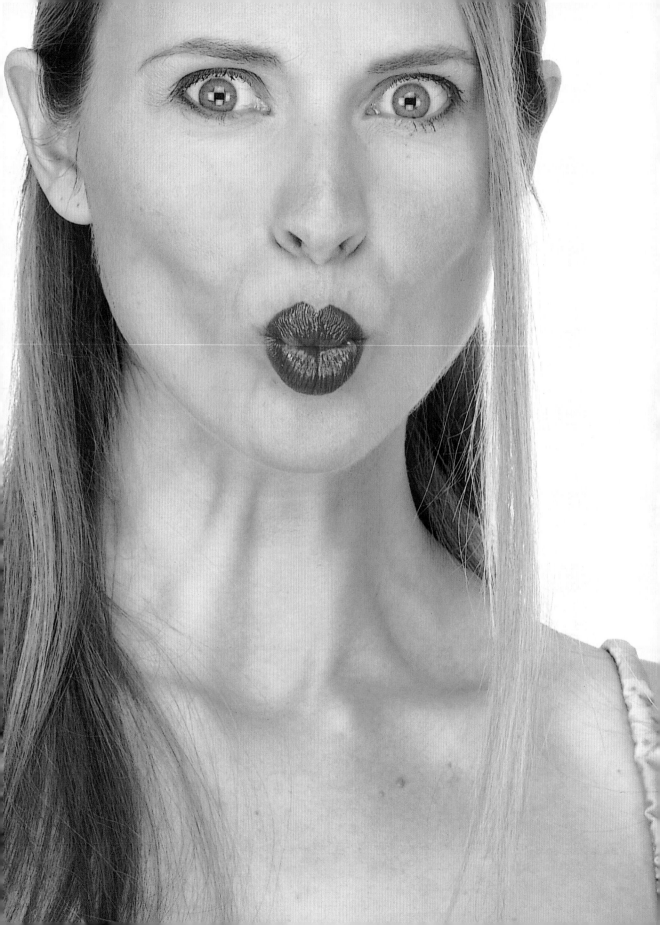

Q+A

■ **I'd love to have a baby, but my partner says he isn't interested. I just know that he'd come around to the idea if I actually got pregnant. Should I just "forget" my contraception and start trying anyway?**

■ **I'm trying for a baby with no luck. I'm getting depressed. Am I infertile?**

● Only if you want him to just "forget" that he ever cared about you in any way. No, of course you shouldn't and you deserve a good slap for even thinking like that. Yes, we've all heard stories of rogues like Warren Beatty who've suddenly gone all doting when their partner gets pregnant but, really, they're in the minority. Instead, the parks are full of lonely single mothers pushing children's swings by themselves. Six words: *Don't get pregnant on the sly.*

So many things need to be in place before you can bring a baby into the world and the relationship is the first. He will *not* be happy. He'll know you've trapped him (yes, he will) and he'll resent you forever. And the child. No, no, no, no, no. Now go off and have a weekend without him to perk his interest back up. Honestly. You girls.

● Probably not. Even though we read countless stories of women failing to conceive, infertility is still relatively rare. Most of us underestimate how long it can take to get pregnant. While some women like Anne (who started this chapter) get pregnant immediately, not everyone does. If it's over a year, see your doctor. If it's under a year, start tracking your periods and be sure you're doing it when it matters.

As for depression, nothing lifts your spirits like a plan. Try this: take folic acid, cut back on caffeine and booze, and quit smoking. Sit on a pregnant friend's bed (an old wives' tale my mom swears by). And, just for fun, say an "Invitation to the Baby." The idea is that babies only come when they're wanted—like men. So find a quiet moment and tell your baby that you are ready for her (or him) and you'd like her to arrive soon. Yes, you feel like a dork doing it. Yes, your partner will laugh at you for suggesting it. But I had a baby nine months after we did it. Good luck.

Don't be scared. You're not the first person it's happened to.

■ My partner says we shouldn't have to "try" to have a baby. He says if it's meant to happen, it'll happen. I know what he means but I'd still like to use proper methods, such as propping my legs up after sex. I'm worried he'll get angry. Help!

● Damn men and their logical minds. Of course he's right, a bit, but there's nothing to stop you helping Nature along. If you want to prop your legs up, ask him to make you a drink after sex. Then do it when he's not in the room. Or run to the bathroom, lie on the floor, and rest your legs up against the bath. I'm not telling you to trick him into having a baby (see Question 1), but anything that makes you feel more optimistic is worthwhile. I wish you well.

■ I had unprotected sex and now I'm worried I'm pregnant. I can't afford a test and I'm too scared to see the doctor. What should I do?

● Take a deep breath. First of all, work out your cycle. Did you have sex 10 to 14 days after your last period started? If not, you're unlikely to be pregnant. Secondly, was sperm actually released inside you? If not, you're unlikely to be pregnant. And lastly, how do you feel? It's confusing, but many of the symptoms of early pregnancy are those you get before a period anyway. They include: tender, sore breasts; heavier vaginal discharge; pains in the lower abdomen; constipation and/or diarrhea; nausea or vomiting.

After you've worked out your cycle and checked your symptoms, if you still think you may be pregnant you must get a test. Either choose a cheap supermarket brand, or visit a health clinic. It's vital you find out as soon as possible. Don't be scared. You're not the first person it's happened to. Whatever happens, you'll get through it.

Whatever happens, you'll get through it.

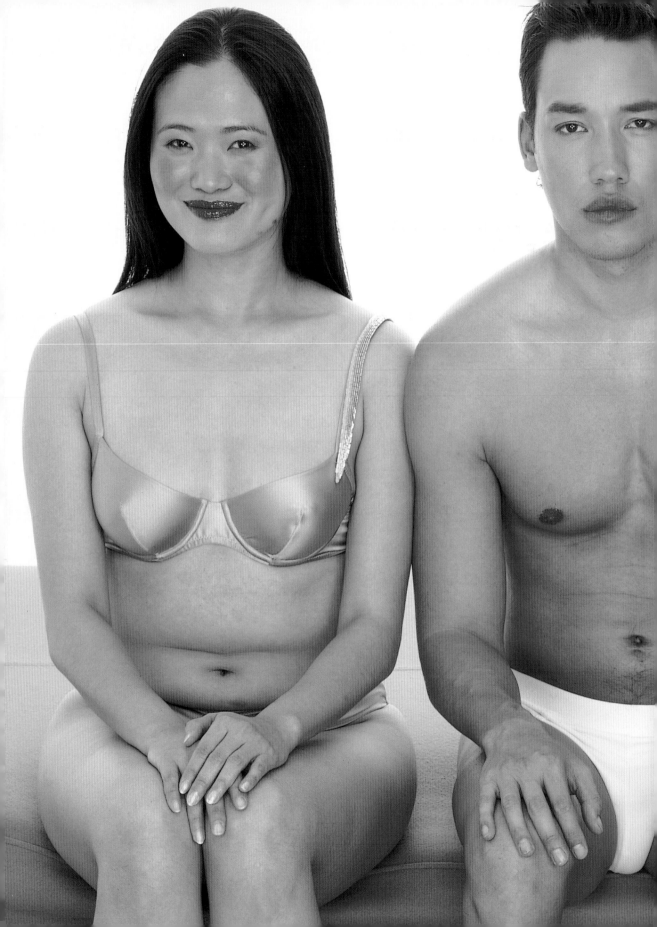

8 Hot monogamy

(how to have great sex for
the first or the millionth time)

Personal story: **Delve into those filthy corners**

Robert and I had been together for seven years. It was getting to the stage when I'd stay up at night after Robert had gone to bed, trying to ensure he was asleep before I got there. I was avoiding sex. Nothing against Robert, but the spark had gone out. We'd always had lovely sex but I was finding it hard to see him as a sexual being. He had become just "good old Robert," and I wasn't excited anymore. One night, he caught me reading a book about men's fantasies. We started talking about it, and he suddenly told me that his deepest fantasy was to spank me. I was so shocked! But as he talked about it, I became curious and out of the curiosity came arousal. It seemed so out of character that "good old Robert" would want to spank me. It made me realize that there were still parts of him that I didn't know about. He regained some mystery and I regained my sex drive.

After that experience, we started incorporating our fantasies into our sex life more and more. Turns out that "good old Robert" had a thing about seeing me dressed up in uniforms (school, nurse, or just even severe work suits). Who knew? Not me! But as soon as I did know, I enjoyed dressing up for him.

It's not fantasy sex all the time, of course. Sometimes neither of us can be bothered. But what it has done is helped us be much more relaxed about admitting what we like. Since he shared his spanking fantasy with me, I feel I can tell Robert anything. That has freed us up to really communicate what we want from each other. It sounds corny, but I really believe we've reached a new level of intimacy. And I'm attracted to him so much more because of that.

Robert 37 and Susie 38

Are you sexy?

I asked that question at the beginning of the book, and I'm coming back to it now. The reason is, that it's very hard to keep the sexiness going in a long-term relationship. If you have children it's doubly hard, but even if you don't it can sometimes seem like the universe is conspiring against you to keep the sexiness out of your life. This chapter will hopefully help you to keep it forever.

There are two main reasons why sex can go off the rails in a steady relationship: repetition and resentment.

Repetition

Do you remember Torville and Dean when they performed their famous "Bolero" routine? (If you don't, it was an award-winning choreographed ice dance that smashed loads of Olympic records.) It was fabulous—all dramatic, intense, with loads of twirling stunts and passion that must have been amazing to perform. The first time. But because it was this famous routine, they had to perform it everywhere. Can you imagine? Doing it over and over …

And let's face it, that's what sex can be like. At the start it's awesome—you can't get enough of each other, you melt when he touches you, his hand on your thigh makes you dissolve with lust. But after a while—yawn. It starts being predictable. You know before you hit the sheets exactly what's coming next (and it won't be

you). It feels like you're following a checklist: Begin with nipple sucking—check. Kissing down his stomach followed by a three-minute penis suck—check. Brief diversion into a 69—check." Argh! No wonder you start redesigning the bedroom color scheme in your brain while he's licking your inner thighs. You can predict every move with an accuracy that a psychic would kill for.

What can you do? All the books say "shake up your moves." But how? Here are five great ways:

1. Opposites attract

Whatever you normally do, do the opposite. This is a great tip for breaking the repetitious cycle and you can start tonight. However you normally begin making love, start the completely opposite way. For example, an ex and I always used to begin our lovemaking with a long slow kiss in bed. Now, he was a fantastic kisser and I'd never deny that those kisses got me going. But *every* time? One night, I grabbed him in the hallway when he got home, yanked down his trousers and gave him a blow job. It ended up with us screwing halfway up the stairs and, well, once the neighbors stopped hammering on the walls, it was fabulous. It broke the cycle. So whenever we started to kiss in bed like we used to, we thought back to the night of the unexpected hallway BJ and remembered there is another way.

A great tip for breaking the repetitious cycle is, whatever you usually do in bed, do the opposite. Try it tonight. I dare you.

2. Reveal your fantasies

This can be a great way to spice up your sex life. Don't keep your fantasies a secret. Most of us fear that our partner would disapprove or even ridicule us if they knew what we secretly thought about. But that doesn't often happen. If you broach the subject with sensitivity—as opposed to grabbing his hand mid-screw, and screaming,—"No no no no no! That does nothing for me. I want you to dress up as a doctor and examine me. That's sexy."—you should find it goes down well.

In fact, when filming *Sex Tips for Girls*, we did a huge section on fantasies. When women revealed their dark thoughts to their mates, the men responded admirably. They took the fantasy as a challenge and were spurred on to recreate them for the girls. One man heard that his girlfriend secretly dreamed about being ravaged by Dracula. Instead of running screaming from the room, he went away and booked a weekend for two at a Gothic hotel, rented a Dracula suit and whisked her away for a weekend of vampiric passion. That could be you. So, share.

3. Flirt with your partner

How do you talk to your other half? If it's degenerated to the stage when you only grunt to each other about doing the dishes, this is the tip for you. It's criminal how some people speak to the person they're meant to love more than anyone else in the world. We're often nicer to strangers in the grocery store than we are to our mates. Well, not any more. Vow, today, that you're only going to compliment your partner for a week. No complaints, no sneers. Imagine he's a friend and speak accordingly. Be positive and supportive. Call him "gorgeous" and "handsome." Be nice. Lay it on thick and see how he reacts. I bet you my autographed copy of *How to Win Friends and Influence People* that it'll re-ignite the fire that's currently smoldering in his pants.

4. Communicate

Sex is the hardest topic to talk about in long-term relationships. It's down to fear—we're scared to bring up the subject in case our lover replies, "Well, to be honest, you haven't done it for me since 1982." If that's you, a clever way to broach the subject is to compliment your partner on everything he is doing right. One night soon, when you're in bed, tell him something he does to you in bed that you really love. (I don't mind what it is and I don't want to know.) Humans are suckers for compliments. He'll probably glow with pleasure and every part of him (yup, even that) will swell with pride. Ask him to do it again. Now his mission will be to recreate that magical moment. Make sure it doesn't backfire though and that's *all* you get.

5. Kiss

What is it about necking? When you meet your

mate, it's all you can do. You kiss passionately as often as you can. It's the most erotic thing ever if you're doing it right. But six months, no, three months, no, one month down the road you barely peck each other. Screw that. Make it your goal to kiss your lover passionately at least once every day. Don't think about it, just do it. Right now. Go and kiss his face off. It's the quickest cure for impotence and sexual boredom ever. You'll feel 16 again.

Resentment

I honestly believe this is the reason why many married women stop having sex with their husbands (or, to a lesser extent, why husbands stop having sex with their wives). Resentment is when you harbor old grudges, piling misdemeanor on top of misdemeanor, without ever admitting them to your mate. Women are more prone to this than men, as we often "let things go" to give the man a chance to make it up later. We're trying to be "nice." Ergo, the "nicer" you are, the more likely you are to be harboring a great big sack of resentment towards your partner.

Does the following situation ring any bells?
Anne and John have been married for two years and recently had a baby. Before the baby, John used to go out every Friday night with friends from work. Now they have the child, he still

does. Anne says, "I try not to mind, I honestly do. But it seems wrong to me that I have to stay home and take care of his child while he's out having fun and pretending he has no responsibilities. I did bring it up once, a few months ago, and John said that if I really hated it, he'd stop going. Of course I felt guilty so I said no. But I only said that hoping he'd stop. He didn't. Now it's getting to the stage where I'm finding fault with everything he does and I can't stand the thought of him touching me. I'm so angry with him, I can't make love with him."

Anne is suffering in silence, which is a one-way ticket to Resentmentville. Unless she stops trying to be "nice" and openly admits that she thinks he's a selfish shit for going out every Friday, they might never have sex again. If you feel you could be harboring resentments, and they're affecting your sex life, what do you do? Here are five things:

1. Don't be afraid to get angry
Think about it, what's going to be more damaging to your relationship—having a one-time big blowout argument, or stopping having sex? It's not the former. If Anne were to scream at John and get her feelings out in the open, they could work something out. But because she's scared of confrontation, she is punishing him in smaller, sneakier ways, like refusing his advances. This is how major problems start. Don't be afraid to get angry. After all, an

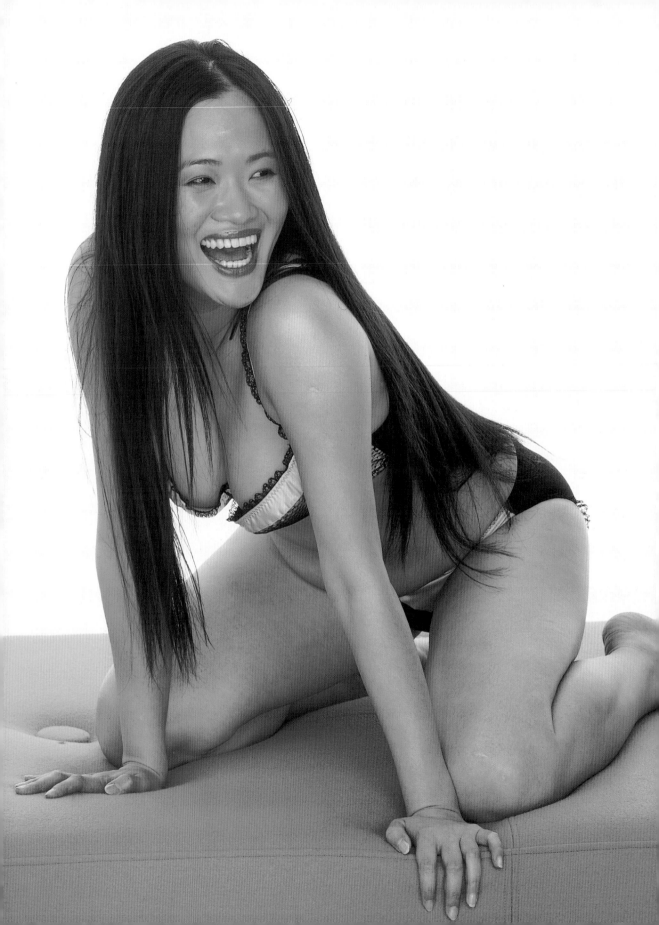

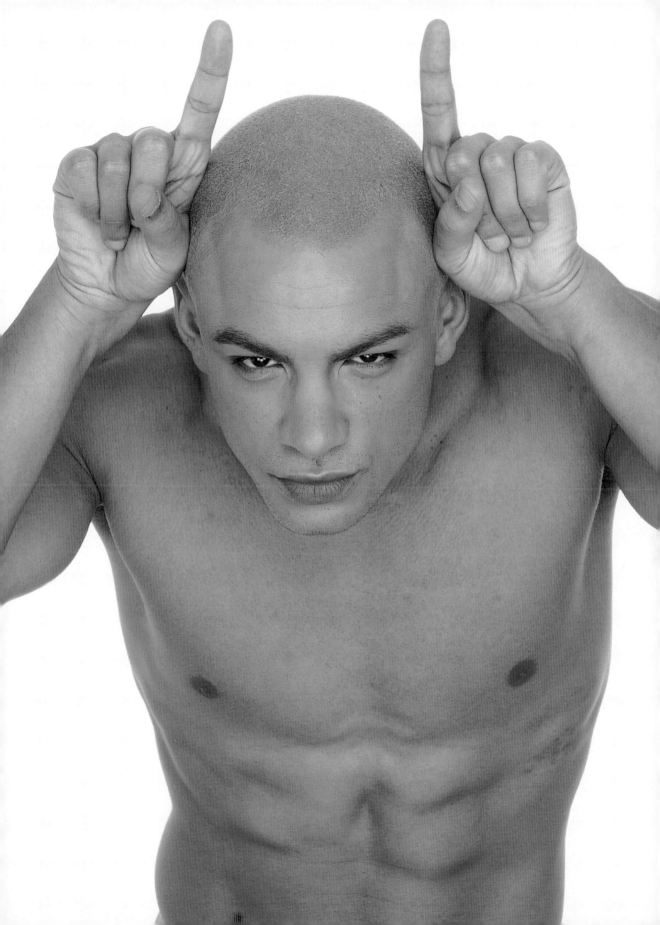

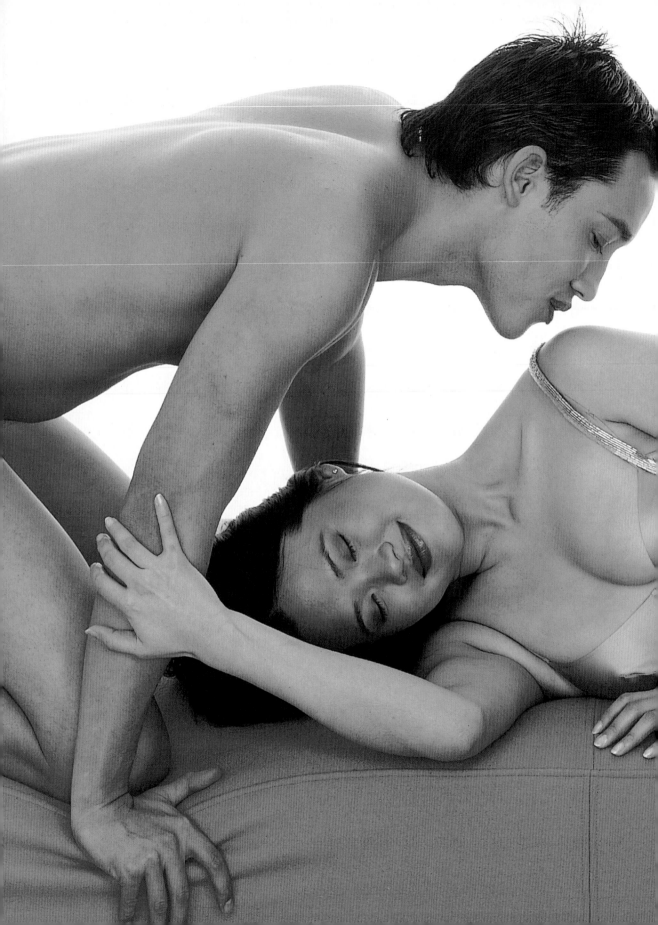

Why stop doing all those sexy
moves you used to love just because
you're in a long-term relationship?
Try flirting and teasing again.
Little kisses all over your partner's
body, feather-light touches,
massages, body painting ...

Girls, don't be afraid to make the first move. When they're in steady relationships, men love to feel wanted. Grab him now. Go on ...

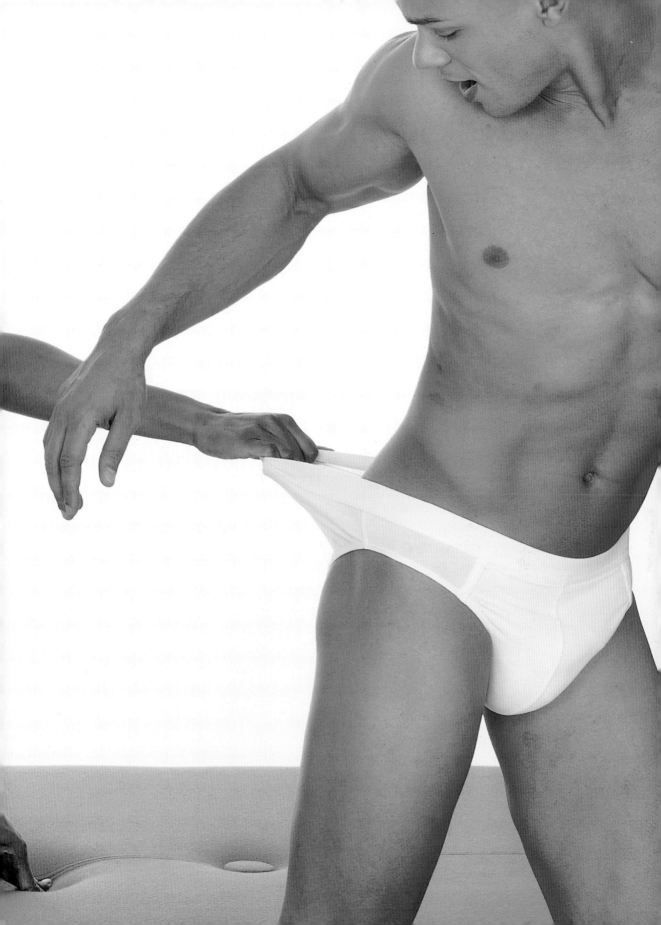

argument can be exhilarating, like having cold water splashed on your face. But slow-burn resentment is like cancer, eating away at your loving feelings until they disappear. Be a bitch, sister. You have my permission.

2. Have your own life

Another cause of resentment is jealousy. Not jealousy of another woman, necessarily, but of interests he has that don't include you. For example, Sarah's boyfriend Tim loves football. Every Saturday he is either at a game or watching one on TV. Sarah is jealous. "I can't help thinking that if Tim really loved me, he couldn't bear to be away from me every Saturday. It stops us doing anything romantic. We can't go away for weekends because he has to watch the game. We never do anything. It's always about football. I'm hurt. I sit there beside him, working myself up into a stew. I've burst into tears at half-time before now."

The important sentence here is: "I sit there beside him." Yuck! Sarah should be out and about, seeing her friends, shopping, or doing whatever makes her happy. By sitting there, getting annoyed, she is building up a whole mountain of resentment. It would dissipate if she just put herself first.

Whenever you find yourself picking at your mate, or trying to change him, it's a sure sign that you aren't busy enough. We often project our feelings of boredom or restlessness onto our partners because they're close by and it stops us having to do the work on us. That's when we start thinking, "If he'd only change X, we'd be so much happier." Nope. You can't change him. You can't change anyone. (Would you want *him* to try to change fabulous *you*?) Get out and get busy and do the work on yourself. If Sarah would stop sitting there beside Tim like Old Faithful, crying into her coffee, he'd be much more likely to treat her nicely.

What's that got to do with sex? Everything. When you're picking at your mate, he'll start to withdraw from you. He wants someone who thinks he's okay. If you don't think he's okay, for goodness sakes dump him and find someone who is! As long as you're picking, picking, picking, he will stop seeing you as sexy and start thinking of you as a surrogate mom. His desire will start to disappear. And the sex will follow.

3. Don't change from a corker to a porker

Another way we can "punish" our partners is by overeating, or just letting our appearance deteriorate. Why? Sometimes overeating is a symptom of serious self-esteem issues. If you think this is you, seek help from a counselor. However, if, deep down, you know that you can control your urges to pig and slob out, your thinking may have gone something like this: "He never compliments me on how I look. He doesn't see me anymore. I could be anyone. Well, screw him, then. If he doesn't notice me, it doesn't matter. I'll have a donut. Ooh, and a slice of pizza. And that pie … "

The truth is, he does notice you. And he notices how well you take care of yourself. If you want him to want you, you must keep up appearances. Paint your toenails. Get your hair trimmed. Watch your diet. Take your makeup off every night. As well as making you look sexier, it'll keep the "edge" in your love life because he won't ever get complacent. If you look lovely every day, he knows that other men will find you attractive. He knows that you'll still have other options and that he can't take you for granted. Beauty is the currency men deal in. They understand beauty. They know that other men want beautiful women.

And, of course, he'll be more likely to want to make love to you.

Also, if you look good, you'll have more confidence. You won't be walking on eggshells, scared to annoy him, if you look as pretty as you can. You'll have more SASSiness if you get wolf-whistled every time you go out and other men flirt with you. You'll remember that you're in your current relationship by choice, and that you can leave if things don't work out. Which, perversely, will probably stop you going.

4. Be happy

I'm not talking about being a fake, Stepford-wife type woman. But if you want your other half to find you sexy and interesting forever, try to be happy as often as you can. Men love happy women. When we're miserable they take it personally. They think they have "failed" if we don't seem glad to be alive, and this puts them off us. Who would you rather make love to—a lover who is upbeat and cheerful, or someone with a long face? If you're fed up, take steps to fix it. And if you're happy, let him know it.

5. From fizzlin' to sizzlin'

These are real-life tips, written by real couples in successful, sexy, long-term relationships. Try a few tonight. Try all of them. Try until you can try no mo'. They're just to give you ideas of fun stuff that will break your routine and start seeing your other half as your sex partner again, as opposed to the man who often forgets to empty the trash.

Blindfolds

Buy a couple of cheap blindfolds from your local costume shop. Cook a romantic meal for your partner, and hand them their blindfold. The idea is that you are both blindfolded while you eat your dinner. Sounds crazy, but it really helps you focus on the sounds and tastes, and it feels sexy too. After dinner, tell your partner that dessert is in the bedroom. Lead each other in there—still blindfolded. Then massage and fondle each other, just feeling your way. We tried this last year and had the best sex ever.
Dan, 33, and Paula, 30

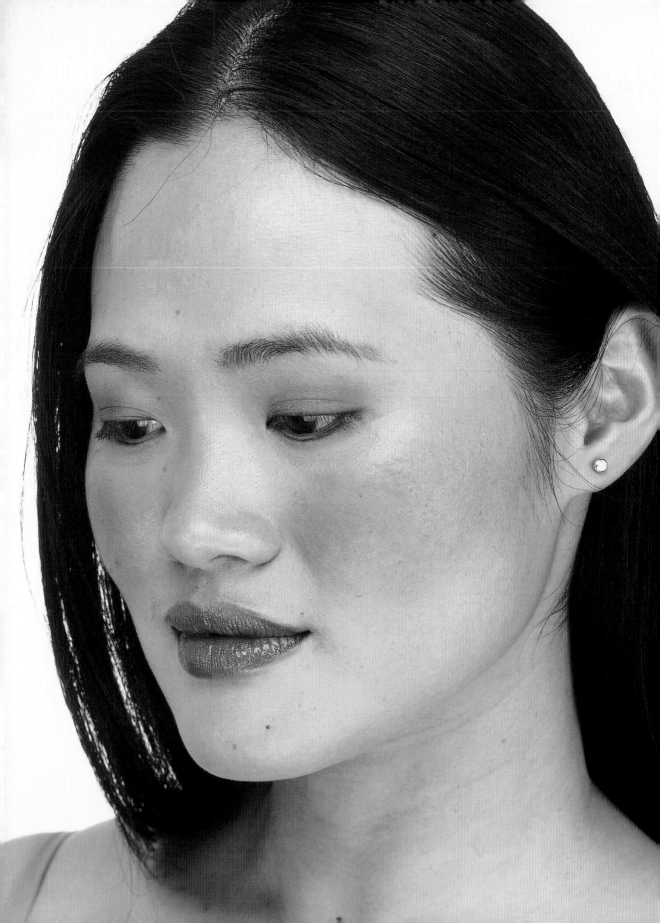

Kissing is the quickest way to rediscover your lust for each other. Sometimes, in fact, it's even sexier than sex. Don't keep giving him "pecks" when you see him—next time go in for a long, hard kiss.

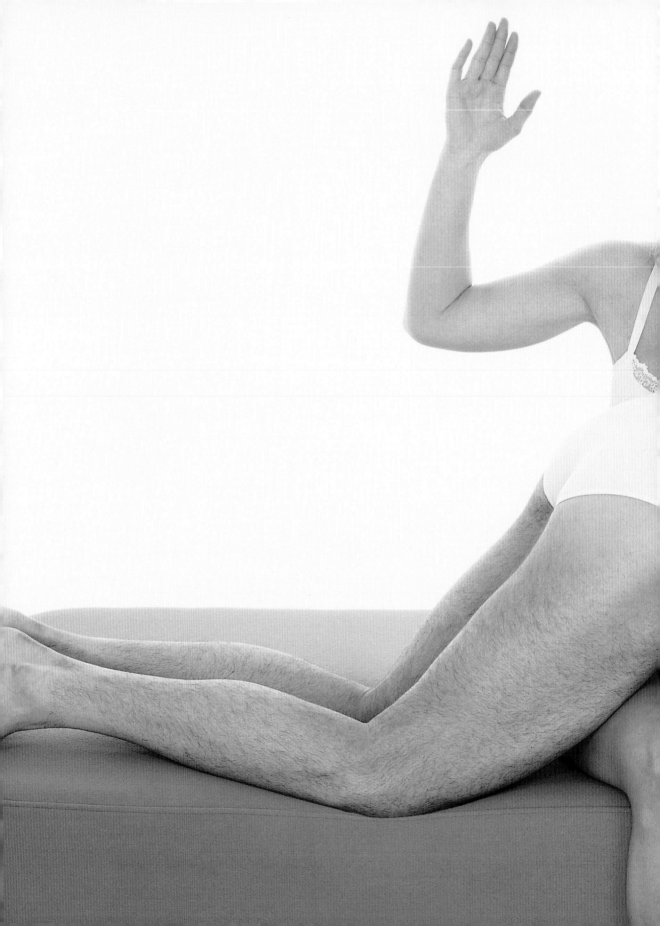

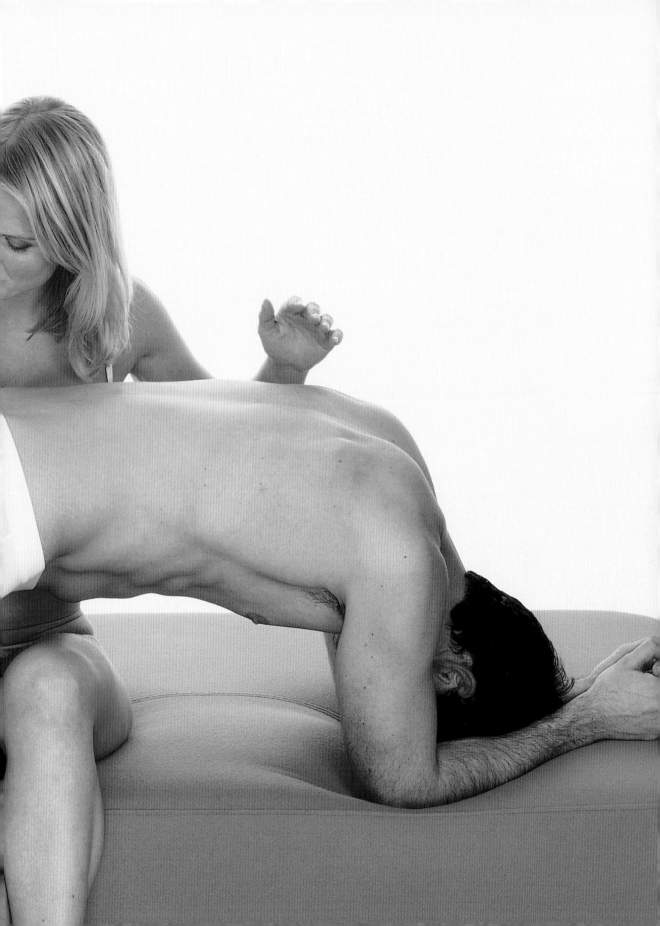

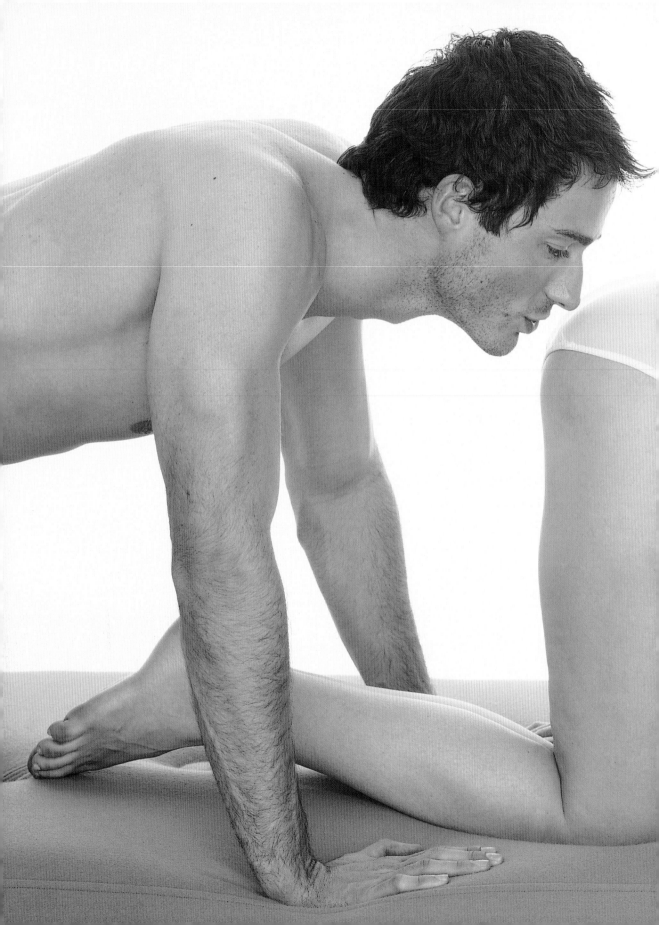

Discover each others' secret desires and have fun while you play.

There are plenty of things you can do to surprise him that will mak you feel like you're 16 again. He'll love you for being naughty.

Doctor love

Borrow a white coat, some glasses and anything that makes you look medical. Tell your lover that you are the doctor and you have to give them a thorough examination to see if they're sexually responsive. Then tell them you have to make love to them as the final test. I love this. Katy, 22, and Nigel, 32

Attend a swingers event

Just go on the internet and type in "swingers." Note what the couples are wearing, then go and buy each other similar outfits. When you get to the event, you don't have to participate if you don't want to. Just tell everyone you're into voyeurism and watch them doing their thing. Then stop on the way home and do it in the car. Awesome. Tom, 39, and Catherine, 40

Do a tantric-sex workshop together

We did this three years ago and still talk about it. Some of the stuff was just funny—like breathing in each other's breaths. But it was sexy just being together and learning new techniques to try. It made our sex life a focus, not just something to be fitted in between work and sleep. Carly, 42, and Richard, 54

Make your own "dirty" movie

Attach a video camera to the bedroom TV, so the picture comes through the screen. You don't have to tape what you do, you can just watch on the TV as you get down and dangerous. Very sexy. We light the room with loads of candles and wear sexy underwear. Peter, 41, and Sasha, 33

Try a sex toy

I bought a vibrator and didn't want Steve to feel like he was being replaced, so we used it for the first time together. He moved it all over my breasts and vagina; I used it on his cock and balls. He really liked it. Now sometimes I start using it before he comes to bed, to warm me up. When he gets into bed, I let him watch what I'm doing. We both find it very sexy. Anita, 33, and Steve, 44

Master and servant

I completely forgot Harry's birthday last year. When I remembered, it was 4:30 pm on the actual day. So, I decided to do something naughty and dress up in a maid's outfit—black top, black miniskirt and a white napkin tied round my waist. No underwear. When he got home I answered the door like I was his maid. Then I wiggled around the living room, cleaning up, taking orders and offering him all kinds of things—letting him get good glimpses of my naked butt. He laughed at first, but I could tell he was starting to get into it. We eventually screwed in the kitchen—with me staying in character all the time. He loved it—his birthday bonus. Tracey, 19, and Harry, 25

Flash cards

This is fun. Get a set of index cards (like you use at work for phone numbers, etc.). Take 20, and on half of them write a body part, like breasts, dick, butt, lips, nipples, thighs, neck, feet, toes and tummy. On the other set write an activity like lick, suck, kiss, massage. Shuffle them up and take turns to play "Snap." You have to do what the cards say to the other person for 5 minutes. Maria, 29, and Steve, 33

Mr. and Mrs.

This is a sexy questionnaire that you do with each other. Write down some questions about sex. Then ask each one aloud, and both of you write down your own answer, and the answer you think your partner will give. Afterwards, compare notes to see how well you know each other in bed. Goofy but kinda fun and it helps you talk about what you like. Good questions are: "What's the quickest way to make me come?" "What's my favorite position?" "What's the best sex we ever had, in my opinion?" "The fetish that most appeals to me is … " "I'd most like a threesome with you and … " Mike, 28, and Lizzy, 27

Hotel sex

Book a hotel room for the pair of you, and take your lover away for a weekend. Before you arrive, package up a sexy "love kit" of nice lingerie, massage oils, a steamy video, champagne, edible body-paints—whatever you think your partner would like. Wrap it up so nothing shows. Give it secretly to the staff when you arrive and have them bring it up to your room as a surprise. David, 45, and Nikki, 43

More sexy surprises

The following ideas are fun, easy ways to spice up your life.

1. Take a Polaroid of your naked body and slip it into your lover's wallet.
2. Write out a "blow job voucher" and give it to him, telling him he can redeem it anytime.
3. Secretly tape a lovemaking session you have, then slip the tape into your lover's car stereo.
4. Answer the door to your mate wearing only plastic wrap.
5. Buy furry handcuffs.
6. Run him a bath, wash his hair and give him a head massage, then "wash" his private parts.
7. Rub vanilla essence or strawberry flavored edible lubricant onto your vagina and tell him to play "guess the flavor." He has three tries— if he guesses right, you do whatever he asks. If he doesn't, he has to pleasure you. Switch afterwards.
8. Buy a furry throw for the bed and some animal-print cushions. See if that doesn't turn him into a tiger.
9. Buy a new perfume and sprinkle a little on the sheets. Have mad passionate sex. Then next time you wear the scent, it'll remind him of that

experience and he'll instantly want a replay.

10. Call him at work and talk very dirty.

11. Send him a sexy text message promising saucy treats for tonight. Then do them.

12. Gather together objects with sensual textures, like flower petals, fur gloves, slippery silky scarves … Blindfold your man and tickle him mercilessly.

13. Start a pillow fight.

14. Frame some erotic artwork and hang it up in the bedroom.

15. Swap the normal bedroom lightbulb for a red one.

16. Prop a large mirror next to the bed. Men love to watch sex.

17. Seduce him in the backyard.

18. Next time you're alone in an elevator with him, see how long you can fondle his penis through his pants before anyone else enters the elevator.

19. Go to a party with him, then tell him you "forgot" to wear underwear.

20. Buy studded condoms. Ask him to try them out.

21. Ask him to tie you up and ravish you. Then switch and repeat.

22. Give him a lap dance.

23. Play strip chess, checkers, backgammon …

24. Watch each other masturbate.

25. Masturbate with a frozen popsicle then let him screw you.

26. Spread honey on his dick then jump aboard. Gives extra friction and feels fabulous. Lick it all off afterwards.

27. Grab him while he's watching TV, unzip his pants and suck away.

28. Give him a massage he'll never forget by covering your breasts with oil and using them instead of your hands.

29. When you next give him a blow job, pull on his toes as he comes. It'll make his orgasm longer-lasting and more intense.

30. Shave off your pubic hair.

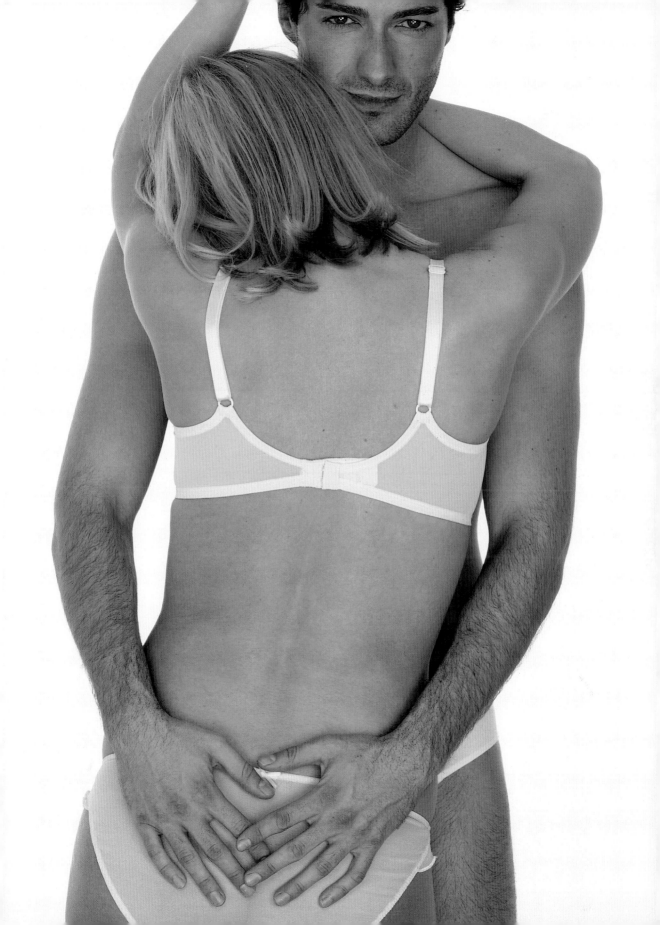

Q+A

■ I love my husband but after 10 years of marriage I've lost my sex drive. He has gained weight since we married and grown a beard. I've tried telling him that I hate his new look but he ignores me. The thought of having him on top of me is unappealing. What can I do?

● Well, a good way to change Beardy Boy back into the man you married is to dig out the wedding photos. Start looking through them tonight, all innocent. Find some nice ones of him and tell him how sexy he looked. Comment that you'd almost forgotten what a handsome, strong jawline he has. Remark with lust on his old lean physique. Then stock the fridge with low-fat food and throw away the junk. If you give him positive reinforcement, he'll be more likely to listen. Then start going for walks in the evenings and ask him to join you. You'll both start shaping up and it'll give you a chance to talk and hold hands again. Good luck.

■ I'm 37, and I've had a few long-term relationships. But every time I'm in one, I want out eventually because I become totally bored sexually. Then I get out of the relationship and back in another one, only to find myself bored again. But then I have this ravenous sex drive for others. This has happened to me enough now that I'm beginning to wonder what's wrong with me.

● You have an intimacy problem. If the sex is good at the start and then you lose interest, my hunch is that along the course of the relationship you find things that you don't like but don't resolve them. If these get pushed below the surface, they could make you resentful or angry. This, in turn, can make you pull back emotionally. If your emotional needs are met, you can actually get more sexual pleasure.

How active are you sexually? Are you open to new things? Do you ever take the initiative? If there's room for you to grow more open, try it.

Does she want more kissing or a different type of foreplay

■ My wife and I have been married for eight years, and we have three beautiful children. Recently, she announced she no longer has passion for me. When we talk, I get the clichéd "It's me, not you" speech. I adore her, but this is putting a strain on our relationship. What can I do?

● It sounds like meeting your sexual needs is one more chore to her. All day long, she's taking care of the kids, then at night, she's taking care of you. I suggest you give her what she needs to feel appreciated and cared for by you. For example, at night, before she goes to bed, just give her a massage or rub her feet without it turning into sex. Give her the message that you understand how tired she is and that she doesn't have to have sex with you in order to take care of you. Also, sit down and talk with her about what turns her on. Does she want more kissing or a different type of foreplay? Find out what's missing and start there.

■ My husband never kisses me. We have the typical peck before we go to work in the morning, but that isn't nearly enough for me. Kissing turns me on, and I have been very direct about that. Even when we have sex, there is never any kissing involved. I've asked him if I have bad breath, and he said no. What should I do to help him want to kiss me?

● Start by kissing him whenever you feel like it. Go to him and don't let him push you away. If he pulls back, look into his eyes and say, "I really want to kiss you." And then just do it and see if he can relax, let go and get into it with you. Show him the power of the kiss and how excited it can make you. When he starts to see the connection between kissing you more and having more intense and frequent sex, he might come around. The key is to show him what he's been missing so that he knows it's not too late to get in on a great thing.

nd out what's missing and start there.

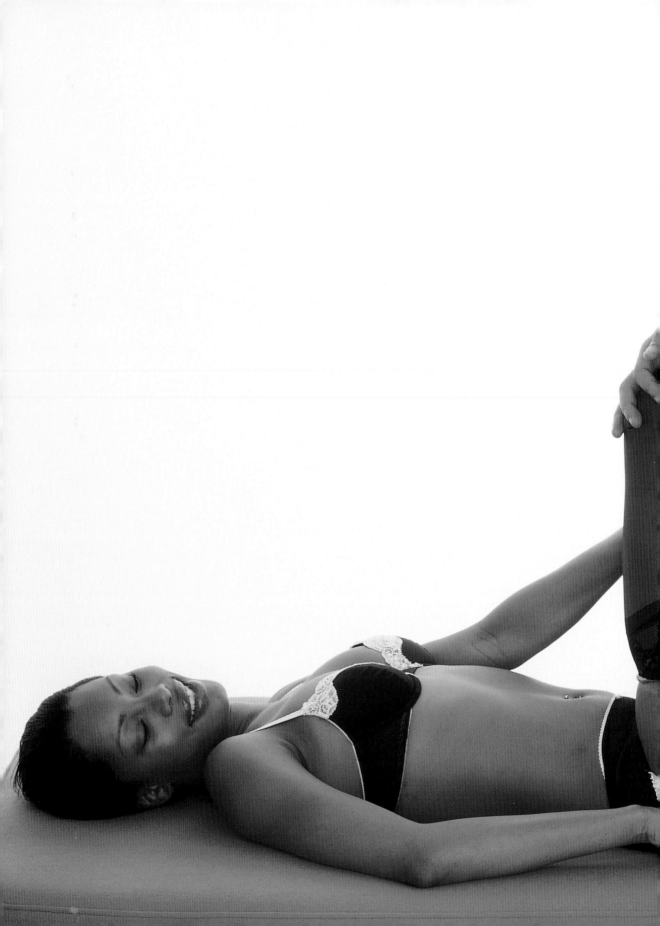

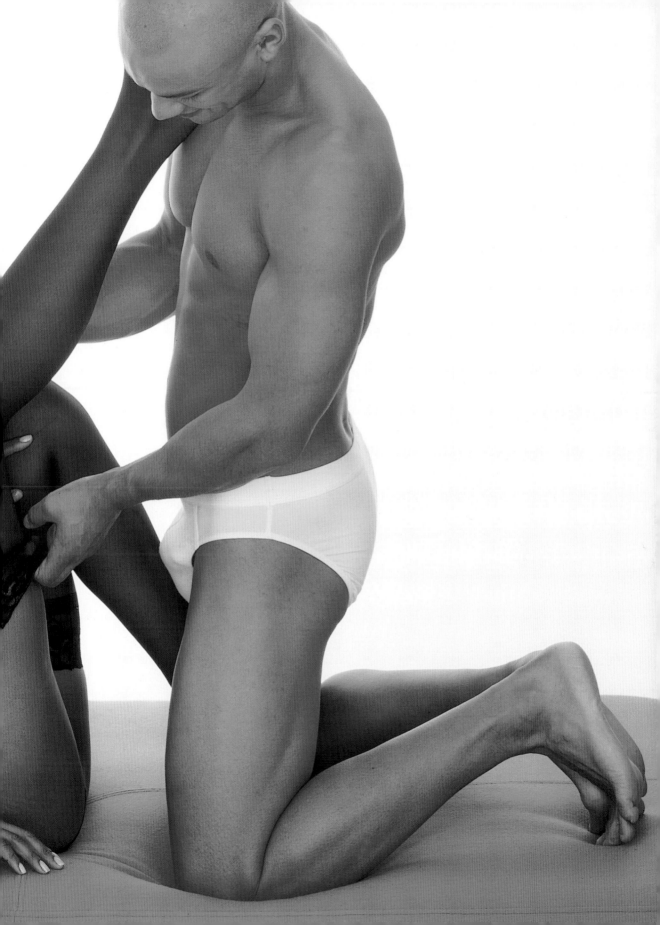

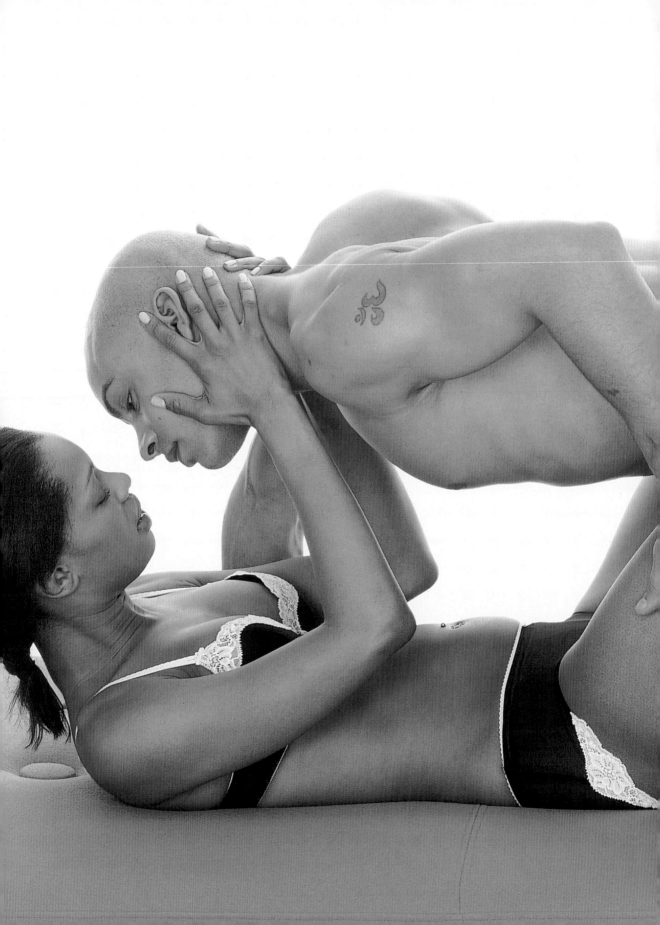

9 Nuts and bolts

Contraception

Contraception is a vital part of a happy, healthy sex life. I'd say it was the most important thing, actually—more important than your blow-job technique, his ability to find your G-spot, even the bounciness of the mattress. It's so easy to forget that sex can get you pregnant, but it sure can, darling. And absolutely the worst thing you can do is have an unplanned pregnancy. If you're ever tempted to skip contraception because inserting your diaphragm or putting on a condom might "break the mood," believe me—nothing will break the mood like the screaming of a newborn baby from beside the bed. Okay?

Enough of the scare tactics. Here come the care tactics. Think of getting your contraception right as the most self-loving, caring thing you can do for your body. You want to be able to have the very best sex life that you can without a painful IUD, badly prescribed Pill or too-thick condom getting in the way.

Choosing the right contraceptive

How do you choose the right method? The best way is to make an informed decision based on all the information and talking to your doctor.

Natural methods

Abstinence

This means not having sex. It's foolproof, but perhaps a bit drastic.

Level of protection: 100 percent.

It's right for you if:

● You're a nun.

Withdrawal

This is when the man pulls his penis out of your vagina before he ejaculates. You don't need any other devices or gadgets at all (except, perhaps, a towel). This is not a method to rely on if an unexpected pregnancy would wreck your life, or if you're worried about a dribble of semen wrecking your sheets. A lot of things can go wrong—the man can get carried away and withdraw too late or not at all; you can get carried away and tell him that he doesn't have to withdraw; he can withdraw in time, but sperm can still be released in his pre-come; he can withdraw and ejaculate outside your vagina, but it runs back in … You get the idea. Also, it offers no protection against AIDS or STDs, because diseases can get passed between you without semen being released.

Level of protection: Around 80 percent.

It's right for you if:

● You're in a long-term relationship and both of you have tested negative for the HIV virus.

● You could both handle an unexpected pregnancy.

● You trust your partner to withdraw at the right time.

● You don't mind the lack of intimacy of his not ejaculating inside you.

Rhythm method

The rhythm method works by charting your fertility cycle so you only have unprotected sex on the days when you're not fertile. You're able to conceive for less than a week every month. This method shows you approximately when that time is. During your "infertile" days you can have unprotected sex; during your "fertile" days you will have to use condoms. To work out your cycle, you can either use a device like Clearblue, which tests your urine, or you can do it yourself. The do-it-yourself method is to chart your cycle on a calendar, marking down the days of your period, and taking your temperature every day. (Your body temperature rises when you're fertile.) It's complicated—you'll need a lot more information if you are going to chart your own cycle—but worth it if you want a natural way to avoid pregnancy.

Level of protection: About 90 percent if practiced correctly.

It's right for you if:

● You're in a long-term relationship where you've both tested negative for the HIV virus.

● You could both handle an unexpected pregnancy.

● You are organized enough.

● Your periods are regular.

● You haven't just come off the Pill or been pregnant (both can throw your cycle off whack).

I want it! See your doctor for full details and all the information you'll need. This isn't something you can fool around with.

Physical methods

Cervical Cap or Diaphragm

These are very similar. Both are rubber discs that fit over the cervix—at the very top of your vagina—and prevent those pesky spermazoids from passing through. For added protection, you use spermicide cream too. You have to get fitted for the cap or diaphragm, which involves an intimate appointment with your doctor or at a family planning clinic. Once you've got your cap or diaphragm, you use it by inserting it before sex and leaving it in place for at least six hours afterwards (although you can leave it in for up to 48 hours if you're planning a bit of a session). You have to stop and insert it—up to two hours before you have sex. Also, some men can feel it up there.

Level of protection: Depends on how good you are at using it correctly; 80-95 percent effective.

It's right for you if:

● You're in a long-term relationship where you've both tested negative for the HIV virus.

● You don't mind stopping to insert it.

● Your partner can't feel caps or diaphragms

(or doesn't get irritated by them if he can).

● You are organized enough to carry it with you everywhere.

● You like the idea of less-messy sex during your periods (the cap or diaphragm can stop a lot of the bloodflow).

● You are happy to insert it yourself.

I want it! See your doctor or a family planning clinic.

Male condoms

You know what these are—they're the (usually latex) sheaths that your partner wears on his penis during sex, to catch the sperm. They are one of the easiest contraceptives to use, just because you don't have to see a doctor: you can simply walk into a drugstore and buy a pack or get them free from a clinic. However, condoms are a pain to put on, and can lessen the sensations of sex for the man and the woman.

Level of protection: 97 percent plus protection against HIV and STDs.

It's right for you if:

● Your man sometimes ejaculates very fast (condoms will help him last longer).

● Your prefer "less mess."

● You don't mind the interruption.

I want it! Buy them at any drugstore or get them free at your local family planning clinic.

Female condoms

Hmmmm … These are an option, but everybody I know who has tried them, hated them. I tested one once for a column I was writing and couldn't get to grips with it at all. It almost flew across the room at one point. However, if you aren't happy with other options, these might be right for you. Female condoms are made of a thin plastic called polyurethane. (This is not latex or rubber, which is good for couples where one or more partners has an allergic reaction to latex.) They are inserted into the vagina, with the solid ring extending outside her vaginal lips, and the man inserts his penis into it.

Level of protection: About 95 percent.

It's right for you if:

● You or your partner is allergic to normal latex condoms.

● Your partner is very reluctant to wear a condom.

● You have multiple partners and want protection from HIV and STDs.

● You don't mind the extra cost—female condoms can be up to three times more expensive than male condoms.

I want it! Try a large drugstore, or ask at your local family planning clinic.

Contraceptive implants

Norplant implants are six matchstick-size rods inserted into the upper arm. No, it doesn't hurt (the nice nurse will numb your arm with a mild local anesthetic). Norplant implants release very small amounts of a hormone much like the progesterone a woman produces during the last two weeks of each monthly cycle. The rods are checked once a year.

Level of protection: Almost 100 percent.

It's right for you if:

● You're in a long-term relationship where you've both tested negative for the HIV virus.

● You are happy to have the rods inserted (and removed).

● You are scatterbrained and/or you prefer not to have to think about contraception every time you have sex.

● You haven't had a reaction to other hormonal contraceptives (like the Pill or Mini-Pill).

● You don't mind irregular periods (these can be a side effect).

I want it! See your doctor.

The Pill

Combined oral contraceptives (that's the technical name for the Pill) are birth-control pills that contain two hormones, estrogen and progesterone. They prevent pregnancy by stopping ovulation and making the lining of the uterus thinner so a fertilized egg can't set up home in there. They're the easiest Pill to take because (unlike the Mini-Pill), you don't have to take them at exactly the same time every day. Perfect for the scatterbrained goddesses among you who like living on the edge a bit. But you still have to remember to take them every day. (Personally, I couldn't be

trusted.) Also, some women report hormonal reactions to it, including weight gain, moodiness and loss of libido.

Level of protection: About 96 percent.

It's right for you if:

● You're in a long-term relationship where you've both tested negative for the HIV virus.

● You don't smoke. There is a risk of thrombosis if you smoke and are on the Pill.

● You suffer from acne. The pill can really improve your skin.

● There are no medical contraindications (a fancy way of saying that you aren't at risk from any medical complications that possibly could occur with the Pill).

I want it! See your doctor or local family planning clinic.

Mini-Pill

Like the Pill, except they contain only one hormone, progesterone. They work by thickening the cervical mucus so sperm cannot reach the egg, and by making the lining of the uterus thinner so eggs can't implant themselves. These are a good option if you've had hormonal reactions to the Pill. The snag is that you have to take them at exactly the same time every day. Ask yourself, are you organized enough?

Level of protection: Almost 99 percent if used correctly (which means they're taken at exactly the same time every day).

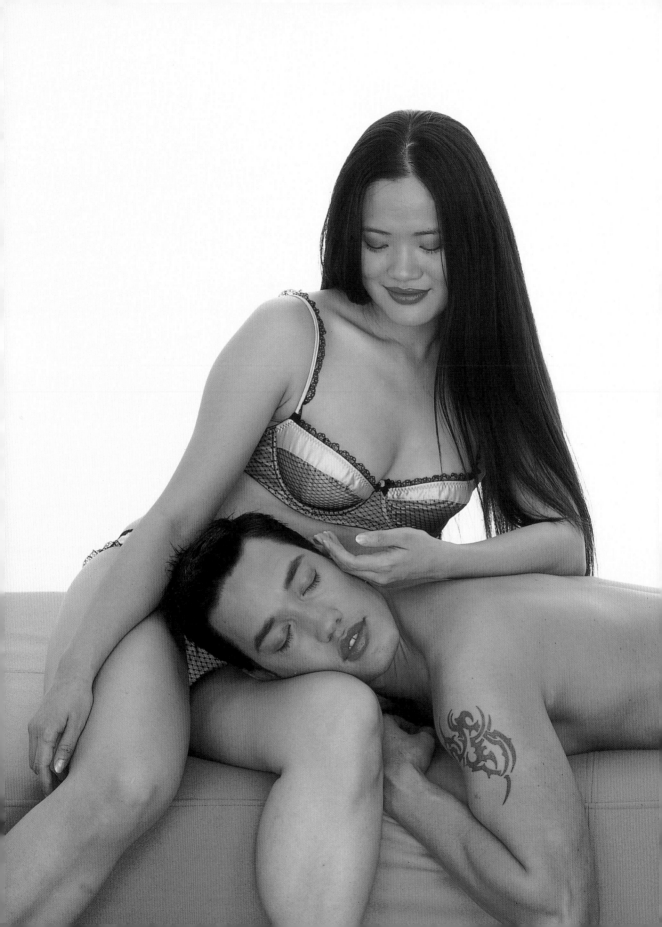

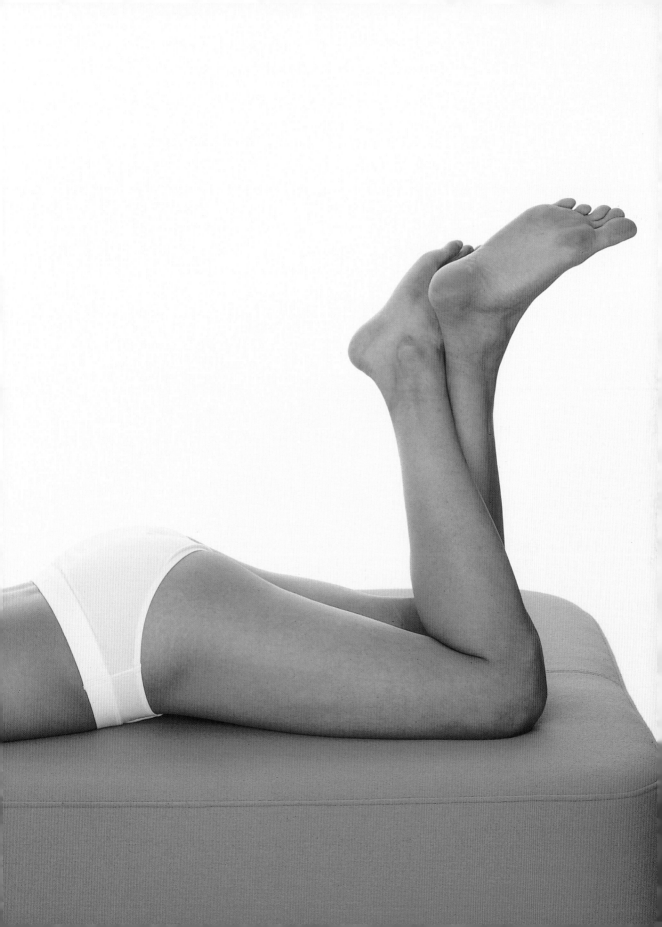

It's right for you if:

● You're in a long-term relationship where you've both tested negative for the HIV virus.
● You're breastfeeding.
● You don't mind irregular periods (the most common side effect).
● There are no medical contraindications (a fancy way of saying that you aren't at risk from any medical complications that possibly could occur with the Mini-Pill).
● You don't smoke.

I want it! See your doctor or local family planning clinic.

Contraceptive injections

How high-tech are these? Contraceptive injections are shots (one every three months) of artificial progesterone, which work by stopping an egg being released. Like the implants, injections are incredibly reliable. Perfect for the more scatterbrained femme fatale, as all you have to do is remember to wander into the doctor's every 12 weeks. However, if you get any side effects (the most common is a very long period that never stops) you're stuck with them for the whole three months.

Level of protection: Almost 100 percent.

It's right for you if:

● You're in a long-term relationship where you've both tested negative for the HIV virus.
● You hate periods—sometimes women stop menstruating after their third injection.

● You're breastfeeding.
● You suffer from PMS, depression or endometriosis (the injections can improve these conditions).
● You don't mind irregular periods (the most common side effect).
● You're prepared for possible weight gain.

I want it! See your doctor or local family planning clinic.

Morning-after pill

Not a regular method of contraception, but good if you've had unprotected sex within the past 72 hours. The morning-after pill is two large doses of the Pill. You take one as soon as you get it, then another 12 hours later. The worst side effect is nausea, which affects half the women who take it.

Level of protection: About 95 percent if taken within 72 hours of sex.

It's right for you if:

● You've had unplanned, unprotected sex within the past 72 hours and need emergency contraception. There's no other reason. These are a big old sackful of hormones; you only want to use them in an emergency.

I want it! See your doctor or family planning clinic immediately.

Permanent methods

Tubal ligation (for women)

Tubal ligation (an operation where the tubes
that carry eggs to the womb are permanently
blocked) is a common method of birth control.
After a tubal ligation, the egg cannot reach
the uterus, and the sperm can no longer reach
the egg. It's foolproof. However, it's permanent.
There's almost no going back. The tubal ligation
operation is much harder to reverse than a
vasectomy, so be absolutely, absolutely sure
you don't want any more kids. The operation is
often performed through a laparoscopy (keyhole
surgery). It's not 100 percent effective in that
if you get pregnant afterward, the risks of
having an ectopic pregnancy (where the egg
grows outside of the womb) are relatively high.

Level of protection: About 98 percent.

It's right for you if:

● You already have children and are
absolutely sure that you don't want more,
or wouldn't ever want more even if your
circumstances were to change (e.g., after a
divorce or death of a child or partner).

● You're in a long-term relationship and both
of you have tested negative for the HIV virus.

● You can handle an operation.

● You don't feel your sexuality will be
compromised by the operation.

I want it! See your doctor.

Vasectomy (for men)

This is an operation that cuts or blocks the vas
deferens, which are the two tubes that carry
the sperm to the penis. It should be thought of
as completely permanent by those considering
it, and not as something that can be reversed
in the event of a midlife crisis. The operation
is a relatively easy one (easier than female
sterilization, for example) and requires no
overnight stay for the man. And, unlike
sterilization, the man can give samples
to check if his operation has been successful.
(They can test the man's ejaculate for sperm.
If none are present then the operation has
obviously worked.)

Level of protection: Almost 100 percent—
but not immediately. The man must expel
15–20 ejaculations to "clear his tubes" of
any remaining sperm.

It's right for your partner if:

● He already has children and is absolutely
sure he doesn't want more, or that he won't
want more if his circumstances change (i.e.,
after a divorce, or death of a child or partner).

● He's involved in a long-term relationship
where both partners have tested negative for
the HIV virus.

● He can handle an operation.

● He won't feel that his sexuality has been
compromised in any way by the operation.

He wants it! See the doctor.

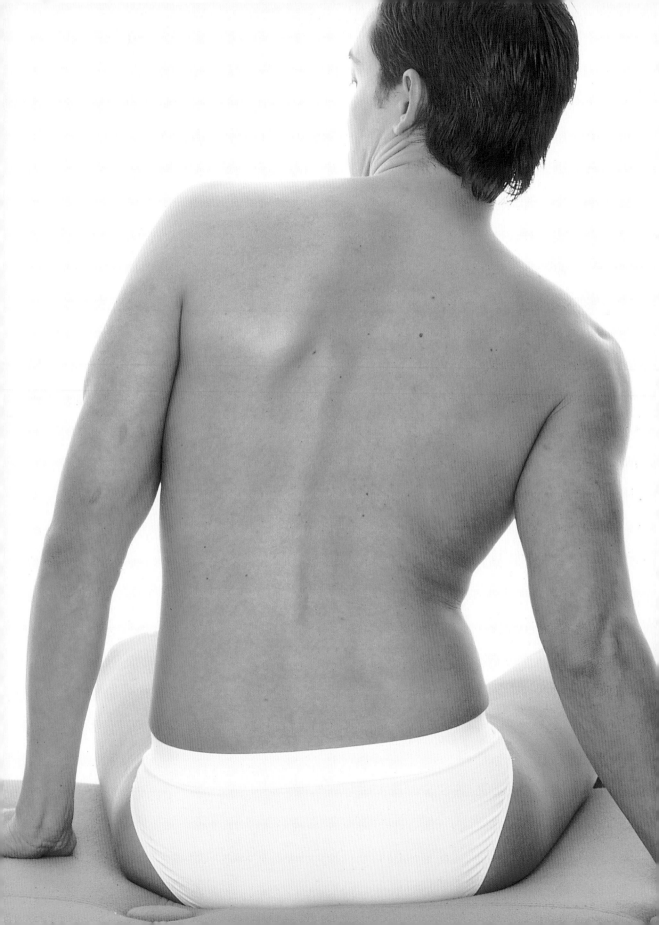

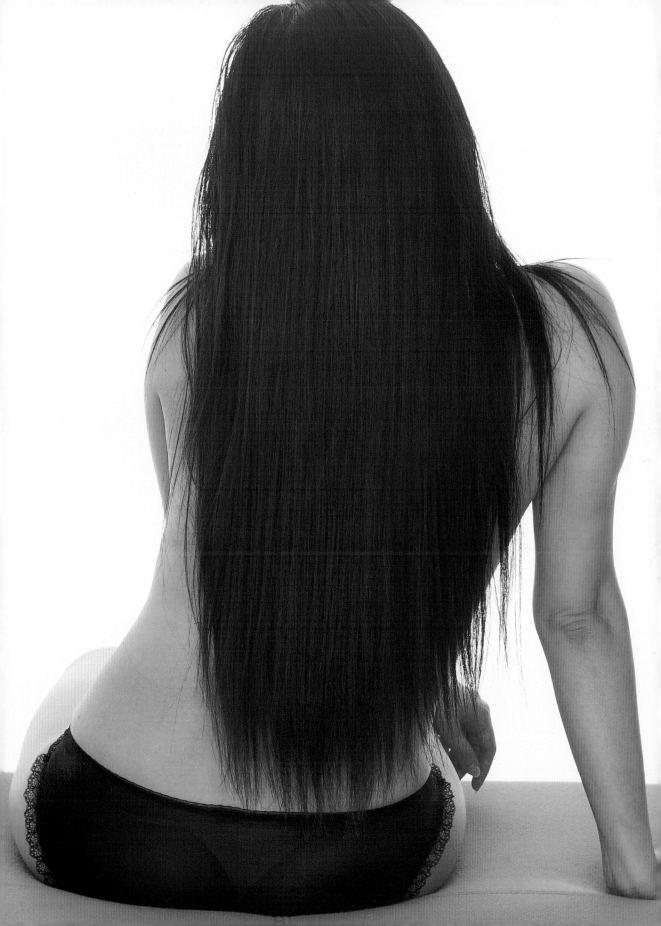

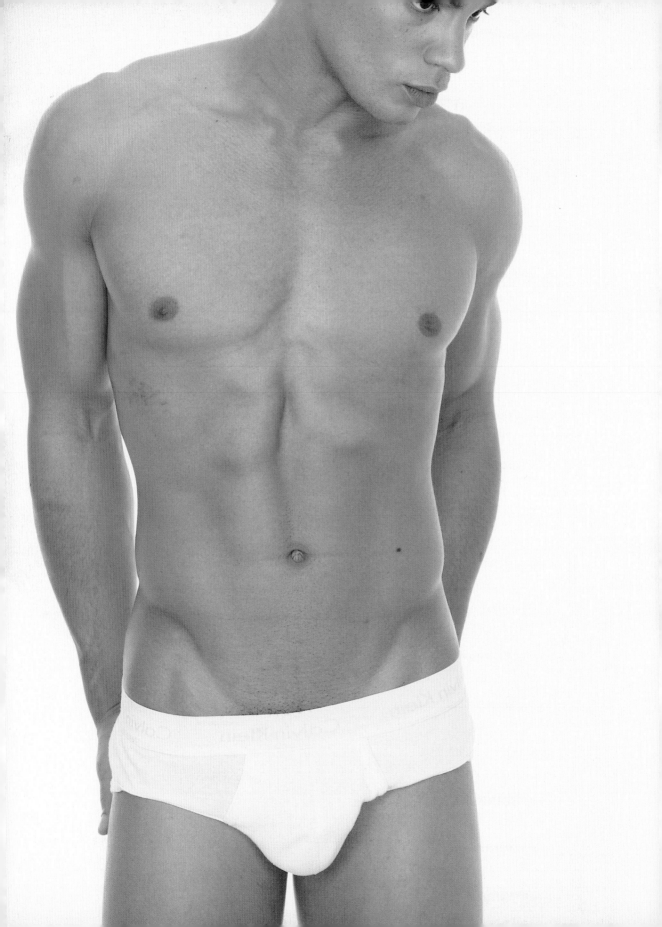

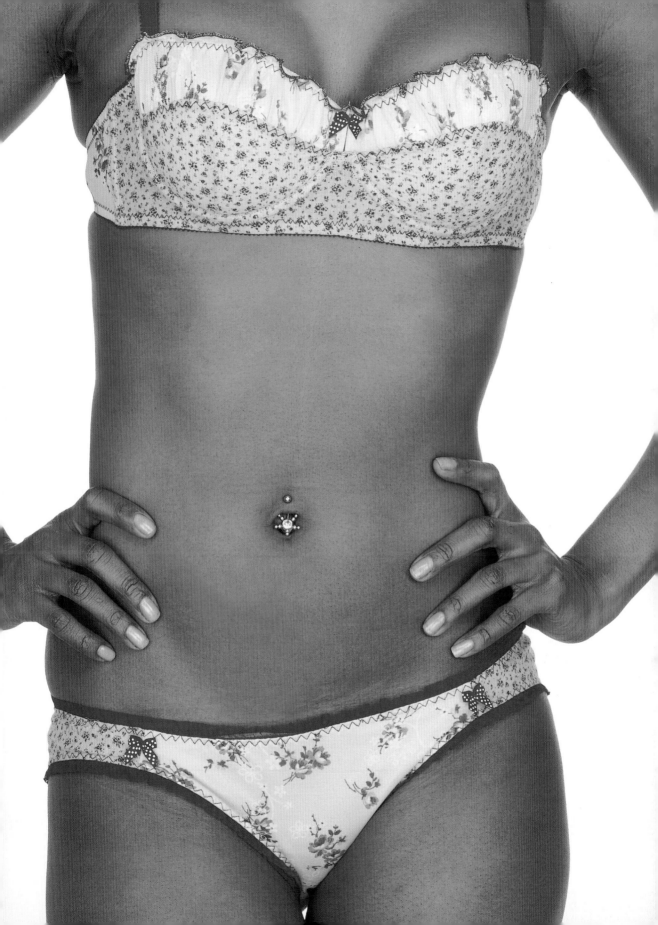

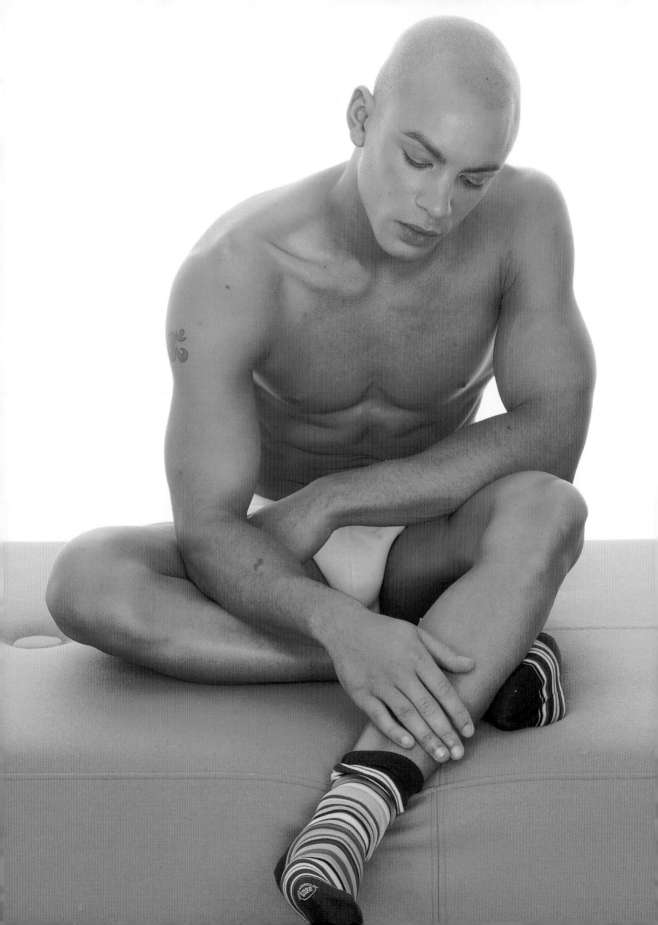

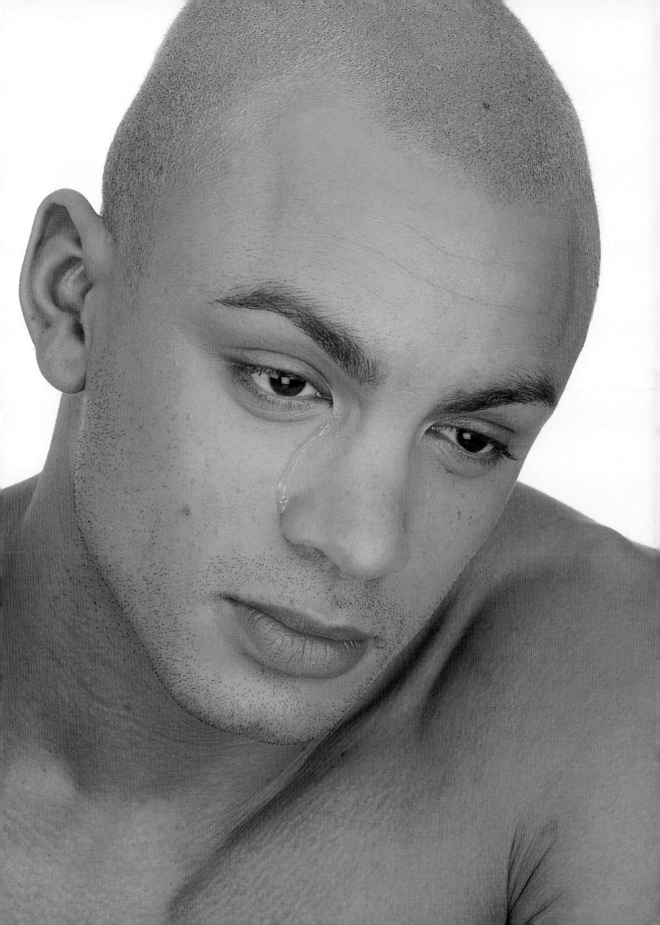

Contraception is a vital part of a happy, healthy sex life

's even more important than your blow-job technique.

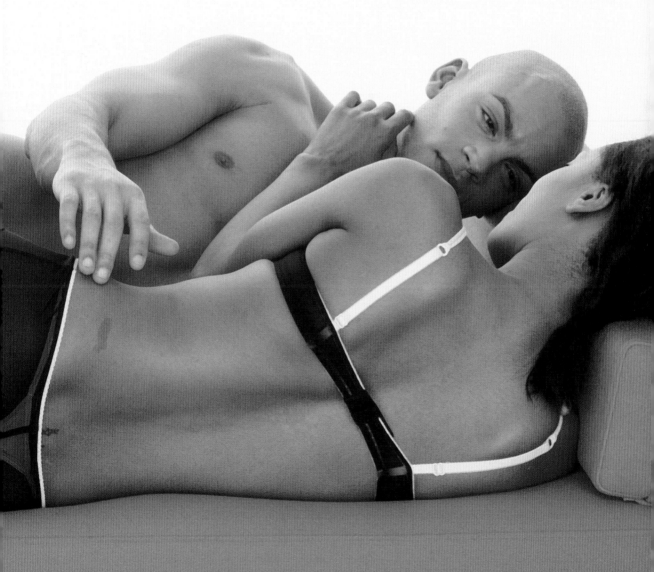

Sexual health

Genital infections and diseases

Below are the genital infections and diseases that are most frequently experienced by women. Some of them and the sexually transmitted diseases that follow them are very common — most of us will experience one or two during our lifetimes. The important thing is not to ignore them. See the doctor and get them treated.

Vaginal dryness

This can be caused by breastfeeding, medicines (including antihistamines), alcohol consumption or a general lack of hydration. Another very common cause is menopause. Occasionally, it can be caused by lack of confidence, anxiety or depression. The treatment is always the same — use a water-based lubricant (like K-Y Jelly or AstroGlide, see page 250 for shopping websites).

Vaginismus

This is where the vaginal muscles tense up, making entry to the vagina impossible. It can happen during sex, or intimate examinations like PAP smears or STD checks. It's a mainly psychological problem, caused by mental issues that make the woman not want to have sex — these could be previous incidents (like rape), lack of trust in the relationship, feelings of low self-confidence … It's a serious condition that will affect your love life to an incredible degree, so see a doctor.

Endometriosis

The lining of the uterus is known as the endometrium, and is shed during the monthly periods. Endometriosis occurs when this lining doesn't pass away through the vagina but gets attached to other internal organs like the ovaries or fallopian tubes. It is a very serious disease that often leads to infertility if left untreated. It also causes incredibly painful periods and raised hormone levels.

BV

Bacterial Vaginosis (BV) is the most common vaginal infection in women of childbearing age. Women with BV may have an abnormal vaginal discharge with an unpleasant odor — some women report a strong fishy smell, especially after sex. There might also be burning during urination or itching around the outside of the vagina, or both. Some women report no signs or symptoms at all. BV can increase a woman's susceptibility to other STDs, such as chlamydia and gonorrhea. Although BV will sometimes clear up without treatment, all women with symptoms of BV should be treated to avoid complications.

Burning Vulva Syndrome

The proper name is vulvodynia. The main symptom is a feeling of burning in the vagina, sometimes after sexual activity, sometimes without any sexual activity. It's often accompanied by vaginismus. If you suspect you have vulvodynia, you'll need to see a gynecologist quickly to get it treated.

Yeast infections

These are painfully common in women. The symptoms are a thick, white vaginal discharge that resembles cottage cheese, sometimes accompanied by an odor and a burning, itching sensation in and around the vagina. There are several over-the-counter remedies that are good, including suppositories, creams and tablets. If you suspect you have a yeast infection, it might be wise to check with the doctor first, just to rule out an STD or BV.

Bladder infections

If you have a constant need to pee accompanied by a burning sensation when you do, see your doctor. It might be cystitis, or it might be something more serious. Drinking unsweetened cranberry juice every day can help. Its acidic content helps change the pH level of your bladder so bacteria can't thrive there, but if it's sweetened, the sugar counteracts the acidity. Bladder infections should be taken seriously as they can lead to worse problems.

Urinary-tract infections

Symptoms are burning sensations during sex and urination. UTIs are very common among women of all ages. Many instances of it could be avoided if women always peed after sex, as they should. Try drinking 12 to 15 glasses of water a day to flush out cystitis—if this fails, the doctor can give you antibiotics.

Sexually transmitted diseases

Any genital symptoms such as discharge, burning during urination or an unusual sore or rash is a signal to stop having sex and see a doctor immediately.

HIV/AIDS

HIV is short for Human Immunodeficiency Virus, which is the virus that causes AIDS. This virus is passed from one person to another through blood-to-blood contact and/or that of bodily fluids including saliva and ejaculate. In addition, infected pregnant women can pass HIV to their babies during pregnancy or delivery, as well as through breastfeeding. HIV infects the cells of the immune system—the very thing the body is supposed to use to fight against germs. Most people who have HIV will eventually develop AIDS as a result of their HIV infection.

Symptoms: Many people do not have any symptoms when they first become infected. Some people, however, have a flu-like illness within a month or two of exposure to the virus. This illness may include:

● Recurring fever or profuse night sweats.

● Headache.

● Profound and unexplained tiredness or fatigue.

● Enlarged/swollen lymph nodes (glands of the immune system), easily felt in the armpits, neck and groin.

These symptoms usually disappear within a week to a month and are often mistaken for those of another viral infection. During this period, people are very infectious, and HIV is present in large quantities in genital fluids.

Treatment: As yet there is no cure for AIDS but symptoms can be controlled or delayed with medication.

Chlamydia

Chlamydia is a common sexually transmitted disease (STD) caused by the bacterium, chlamydia trachomatis, which can damage a woman's reproductive organs. Even though symptoms of chlamydia are usually mild or absent, serious complications that cause irreversible damage, including infertility, can occur "silently" before a woman ever recognizes a problem. Chlamydia can also cause discharge from the penis of an infected man.

Symptoms: Chlamydia is known as a "silent" disease because about three-quarters of women infected and about half of infected men have no symptoms. Women who have symptoms might have an abnormal vaginal discharge or a burning sensation when urinating. When the infection spreads from the cervix to the fallopian tubes, some women still have no signs or symptoms; others have lower abdominal pain, low back pain, nausea, fever, pain during intercourse, or bleeding between menstrual periods. Chlamydial infection on the cervix can spread to the rectum.

Treatment: Antibiotics.

Genital herpes

Genital herpes is caused by the herpes simplex viruses.

Symptoms: Most individuals only display minimal symptoms. They typically appear as blisters on or around the genitals or anus. Blisters can be inside the vagina and go unnoticed. The blisters break, leaving tender ulcers. Typically, another outbreak can appear weeks or months after the first, but it is almost always less severe and shorter than the first. Although the infection can stay in the body indefinitely, the number of outbreaks tends to decrease over a period of years.

Treatment: Antibiotics and antiviral medication. Women with an active genital herpes lesion cannot deliver their baby vaginally.

Gonorrhea

Gonorrhea is a common sexually transmitted disease. Gonorrhea is caused by neisseria gonorrheae, a bacterium that can grow and multiply easily in the warm, moist areas of the reproductive tract, including the cervix, womb, and fallopian tubes in women, and in the urethra in women and men. The bacterium can also grow in the mouth, throat, eyes, and anus.

Symptoms: In women, the symptoms are often mild, and many women display no symptoms at all. The initial symptoms include a painful or burning sensation when urinating, increased vaginal discharge, or vaginal bleeding in between periods.

Treatment: Antibiotics.

Genital HPV infection

Genital HPV infection is caused by human papillomavirus (HPV), a group of viruses that includes more than 100 different strains. Some of these viruses are called "high-risk," and may cause abnormal smear tests. They may also lead to cancer. Others are called "low-risk" types, and they may cause mild smear-test abnormalities or genital warts. Genital warts are single or multiple growths or bumps that appear in the genital area.

Symptoms: Most people who become infected with HPV will not have any symptoms and the infection will clear on its own.

Treatment: In most women the infection goes away on its own. The treatments provided are directed to the changes in the skin or mucous membrane caused by HPV infection, such as warts and precancerous changes in the cervix.

Syphilis

Syphilis is caused by the bacterium treponema pallidum. It has often been called "the great imitator" because so many of the signs and symptoms are indistinguishable from those of other diseases.

Symptoms: Many women infected with syphilis do not have any symptoms for years, yet remain at risk if they are not treated. Men are easier to diagnose.

Treatment: Penicillin.

Trichomoniasis

Trichomoniasis is a common sexually transmitted disease that affects women and men, although symptoms are more common in women.

Symptoms: Many women have symptoms that include a frothy, yellow-green vaginal discharge with a strong odor. The infection also may cause discomfort during sex and urination, as well as irritation and itching around the genitals. In rare cases, lower abdominal pain can occur. Symptoms usually appear within 5 to 28 days of exposure.

Treatment: The prescription drug Metronidazole, given by mouth in a single dose.

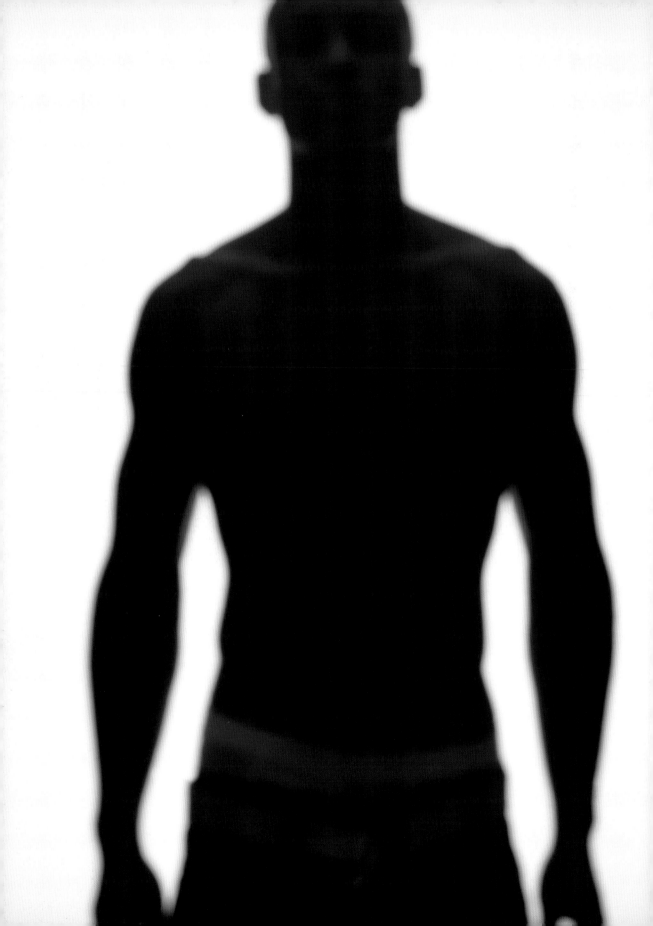

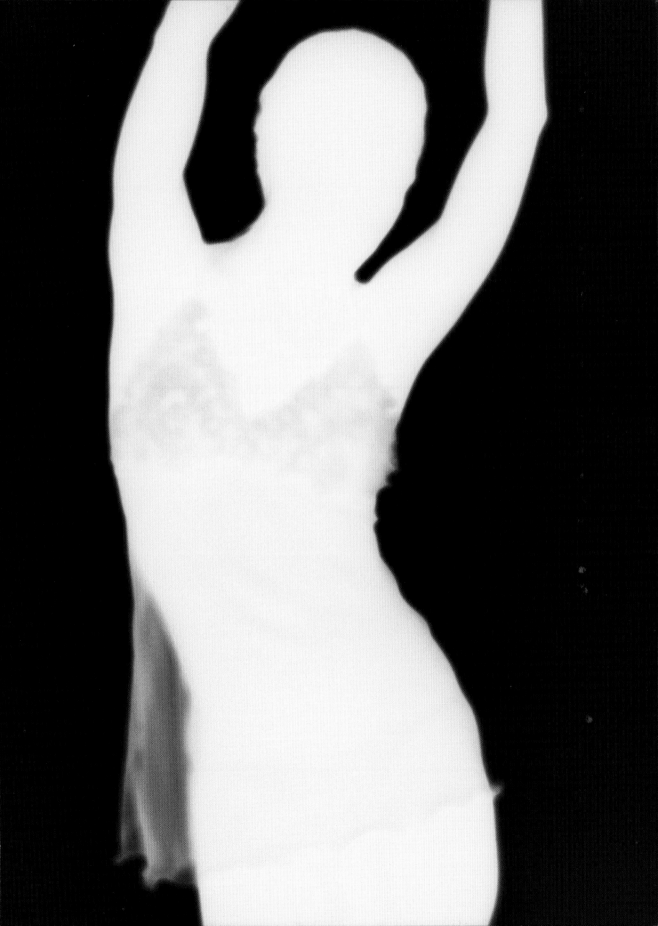

Useful resources

Anderson, Dan and Berman, Maggie *Sex Tips for Straight Women from a Gay Man*, Regan Books, 1997
Everett, Flic *Sex Tips for Girls*, Channel 4 Books, 2002
Everett, Flic *How to be a Sex Goddess*, Carlton Books, 2004
Godson, Suzi *The Sex Book*, Cassell Illustrated, 2002
Paget, Lou *365 Days of Sensational Sex*, Gotham Books, 2003
Paget, Lou, *How to Give Her Absolute Pleasure: Totally Explicit Techniques Every Woman Wants Her Man to Know*, Broadway, 2000
Paget, Lou *How to be a Great Lover*, Broadway, 1999
Paget, Lou *The Big O: How to Have Them, Give Them, and Keep Them Coming*, Broadway, 2001
St. Claire, Olivia *203 Ways to Drive a Man Wild In Bed*, Harmony, 1993
Taylor, Kate *The Good Orgasm Guide,* Barnes & Noble, 2003
Taylor, Kate *Life's Too Short for Tantric Sex,* Marlowe & Co, 2003

Information websites and directories:

www.goaskalice.columbia.edu
www.howtohavegoodsex.com
www.sexinfo101.com
www.women.com
www.babeland.com/sexinfo
www.mypleasure.com/education
www.sexuality.about.com
www.bettersex.com
dir.yahoo.com/Society_and_Culture/Sexuality

Shopping websites:

www.babeland.com
www.mypleasure.com
www.goodvibes.com
www.libida.com
www.extracurious.com
www.spicygear.com
www.grandopening.com
www.venusenvy.ca (Canada)
www.comeasyouare.com (Canada)

Index

Thanks to ...

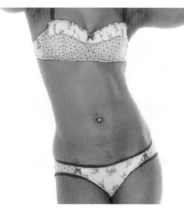

Betsy wore Agent Provocateur

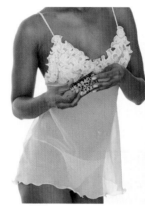

Betsy wore Myla

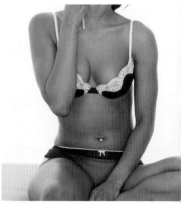

Betsy wore Marks and Spencer

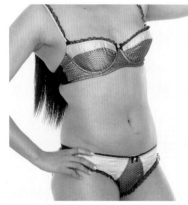

Mei wore Marks and Spencer

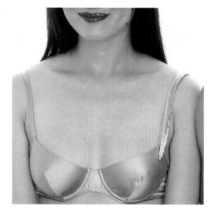

Mei wore Myla

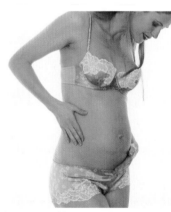

Lynne wore Marks and Spencer

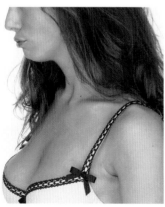

Serena wore Marks and Spencer

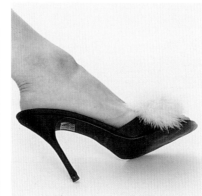

Shoes by Agent Provocateur

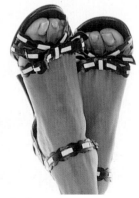

Shoes by Agent Provocateur

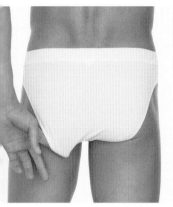

guys wore underwear by Marks & Spencer

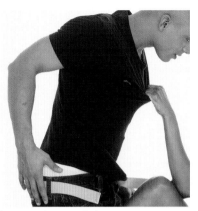

Lee wore his own clothes

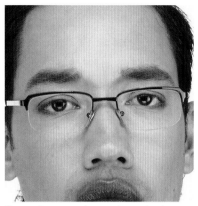

Christopher wore the art director's glasses

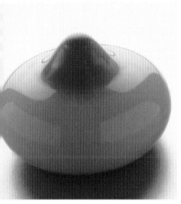

s by Myla

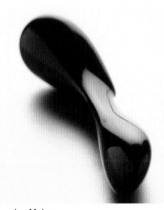

Toys by Myla

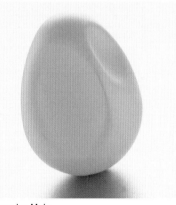

Toys by Myla

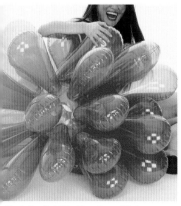

Chair by Eat My Handbag Bitch

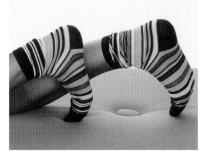

Socks from the collection of Simon Wilder